Snoring and Sleep Apnea

SLEEP WELL, FEEL BETTER

FOURTH EDITION

Snoring and Sleep Apnea

SLEEP WELL, FEEL BETTER

Ralph A. Pascualy, MD

FOURTH EDITION

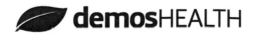

Visit our web site at www.demosmedpub.com

Illustrations: Robert Holmberg, University of Washington, Health Sciences Center for Educational Resources.

Photographs: The following images were used with permission from ®ResMed Corporation, 2007: S8 Elite with humidifier, S8 Escape, and C-Series Tango.

Library of Congress Cataloging-in-Publication Data
Pascualy, Ralph A., 1951–
    Snoring and sleep apnea: sleep well, feel better / Ralph A. Pascualy. – 4th ed.
      p. cm.
    ISBN-13: 978-1-932603-26-2 (pbk. : alk. paper)
    ISBN-10: 1-932603-26-3 (pbk. : alk. paper)
    1. Sleep apnea syndromes–Popular works.   2. Snoring–Popular works.   I.Title.
    RC737.5.P37 2008
    616.2'09—dc22
                            2007047889

SPECIAL DISCOUNTS ON BULK QUANTITIES of Demos Medical Publishing books are available to corporations, professional associations, pharmaceutical companies, health care organizations, and other qualifying groups. For details, please contact:

Special Sales Department
Demos Medical Publishing
386 Park Avenue South, Suite 301
New York, NY 10016
Phone: 800–532–8663 or 212–683–0072
Fax: 212–683–0118
E-mail: orderdept@demosmedpub.com

Made in the United States of America

07 08 09 10 5 4 3 2 1

Contents

Foreword

Sleep apnea syndrome is number one among the hundred-plus sleep disorders recognized today. Why?

1. Sleep apnea is common: it affects one in ten middle-aged men. It is slightly less common in women.
2. Sleep apnea, untreated, can be deadly.
3. Sleep apnea patients are poorly diagnosed and treated because of the lack of trained sleep experts.

Sleep apnea robs people of vitality, health, and sometimes life itself. Loss of vitality will be familiar to many readers of this book. People suffering from sleep apnea fall asleep anywhere and everywhere, even while driving. Their heavy snoring disrupts their own sleep and often that of their family. They drag themselves to work despite exhaustion, doze at their desks, stumble home completely drained, and fall asleep on the sofa. They lack the energy to enjoy family life or the company of friends.

The health consequences of sleep apnea are even more grave. Untreated sleep apnea puts people at high risk for driving accidents, high blood pressure, stroke, irregular heart rhythms, and other life-threatening complications.

Treatment is available and dramatically effective. Formerly sick, sleepy people quickly regain their vigor, resume their cherished activities, and thrive. Life is restored.

Accurate diagnosis is the major problem. Eighty to ninety percent of sleep apnea victims are undiagnosed. The National Commission on Sleep Disorders Research has heard countless testimonies of patients suffering for 10 years or more before sleep apnea was correctly diagnosed and treated.

My primary mission in life today is to lift the shroud of darkness surrounding sleep disorders, and with it years of prolonged and needless suffering. Education is the key— public education, patient education, and medical education.

This new edition of *Snoring and Seep Apnea* answers all three of those educational needs. It educates the sleep apnea sufferer and the public alike. Further, this book is an authoritative survey of sleep apnea diagnosis and treatment for the primary care physician.

This book is an excellent guide for people who suspect they have sleep apnea, for people who have been diagnosed, and for those undertaking lifelong treatment.

I recommend this book to all those with sleep apnea and their friends and families. Use it as a pathfinder. Let it point the way out of the twilight of sleep apnea to timely diagnosis, appropriate treatment, and a bright future.

William C. Dement, MD, PhD
Lowell W. and Josephine Q. Berry
Professor of Psychiatry and Behavioral Sciences
Stanford University School of Medicine
Division Chief
Stanford University Division of Sleep
Palo Alto, California

Preface

Sleep apnea is now recognized as a common and major medical disorder that can significantly impact cardiovascular and mental health, driving safety, and day-to-day functions at home and work. There are over 4,000 sleep centers across the United States and sleep medicine has been recently recognized by organized medicine as a real sub-specialty. Yet millions of individuals continue to suffer without care for their sleep disorder or receive sub-standard treatment and feel dejected that their condition has not improved.

The Main Challenge

This book will help you choose the most appropriate treatment for your problem whether it be surgical, dental, or medical intervention rather than using a CPAP machine. Nevertheless, we know that CPAP therapy continues to be the most common and effective long-term therapy. Why is it then that perhaps half of all patients prescribed a CPAP device are not using it effectively? The current model of care for sleep apnea is focused around the diagnosis and the initial treatment. But for most patients sleep apnea is a chronic and life-long problem that requires a chronic disease model of long-term care. Unfortunately, the health care system provides incentives for the initial diagnosis and treatment, but very little to assist patients in staying compliant with necessary care. This is the great challenge facing the field today and until effective care systems are in place individual patients will face significant challenges obtaining the care they need.

What This Book Will Do for You

More than ever, patients need to be well-informed consumers and ready to be assertive about receiving the appropriate diagnostic tests and the most effective treatments.

The information in this book will enable you to become an effective consumer and find relief from snoring and sleep apnea.

The beginning of the book describes the causes and consequences of sleep apnea, the tests for diagnosing sleep apnea, and pros and cons of current treatments.

Chapter 12 tells how to find a qualified sleep specialist and the nearest accredited sleep testing center.

Chapters 13 through 15 contain suggestions about living with sleep apnea and dealing with the treatment process, plus information on products and services for people who are being treated for sleep apnea.

The names of patients have been changed to preserve their privacy. In the interest of simplicity and because sleep apnea is more common among males, patients usually have been referred to as "he" and their partners as "she." This should not be interpreted to imply any disregard for the many women who have sleep apnea and are under diagnosed for the very reason that this problem has incorrectly been considered a male disorder.

You can free yourself from the twilight world of lifeless days and broken nights.

Ralph A. Pascualy, MD

Acknowledgments

I am grateful to three of my colleagues in the practice of sleep disorders medicine for their time, expertise, and cogent suggestions for this Fourth Edition:

Dr. Darius Rhodes-Zoroufy, of the American Board of Sleep Medicine: Chapters 1–15. Dr. Preetam Bandla of the American Board of Sleep Medicine a specialist in pediatric sleep disorders: Chapters 12 and 13. John Basile, manager of ProCPAP Solutions, and a specialist in CPAP therapy: Chapters 17 and 18.

Finally, Sally Warren Soest, the coauthor of previous additions. I am grateful for her dedication to the education and support of sleep apnea patients, and for her time, research, and work in revising and updating material for this new edition.

Do You Have Sleep Apnea?

The top 10 symptoms of sleep apnea:

1. Loud, irregular snoring, snorts, gasps, and other unusual breathing sounds during sleep
2. Long pauses in breathing during sleep
3. Excessive daytime sleepiness
4. Fatigue
5. Obesity
6. Changes in alertness, memory
7. Changes in mood, personality, or behavior
8. Impotence
9. Morning headaches
10. Bed-wetting

Untreated sleep apnea can cause 12 serious medical problems:

1. Twenty times greater risk of heart attack
2. Three times greater risk of stroke
3. Fifteen times higher risk of automobile wrecks and workplace accidents
4. Irregular heartbeat
5. Increased risk of heart failure
6. High blood pressure
7. Excessive sleepiness
8. Impotence
9. Uncontrollable weight gain
10. Psychological symptoms, such as irritability and depression
11. Deterioration of memory, alertness, and coordination
12. Death

What Is Sleep Apnea?

Sleep apnea (The word *apnea* comes from the Greek prefix *a* ["no"] and the Greek word *pnoia* ["breath"]. It is pronounced AP-nee-uh.) is a breathing disorder that affects people while they sleep, usually without their knowing it. The most common symptom is loud, heavy snoring, which is often treated as a joke. But sleep apnea is no joking matter. Sleep apnea is a potentially fatal disorder. It can often result in heart problems, automobile accidents, strokes, and death.

People with sleep apnea stop breathing repeatedly during a night's sleep. Breathing may stop 10, 20, or even 100 or more times per hour of sleep and may not start again for a minute or longer. As you can imagine, these sleep/breathing disruptions deprive the person of both sleep and oxygen.

"So what?" you may think. "I'm a little tired or sleepy during the day. Why should this be considered a medical problem?"

There are actually two problems. The first is that sleep apnea is a serious health hazard. It is one of the top four causes of cardiovascular disease, along with obesity, diabetes, and smoking.

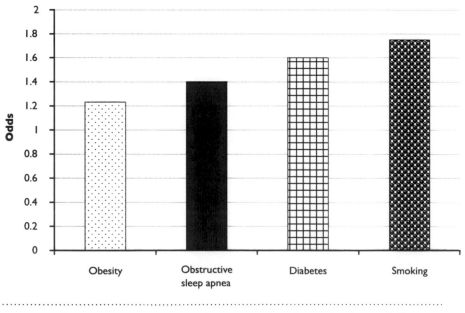

Sleep apnea is among the top four causes of cardiovascular disease (1,2).

The second medical problem with sleep apnea is that an alarming number of people have it and don't know it — between 20 million and 25 million Americans. In a recent study of 30 to 60 year olds, 24 percent of the men and 9 percent of the women had signs of sleep apnea (see chart at the top of the next page) (3).

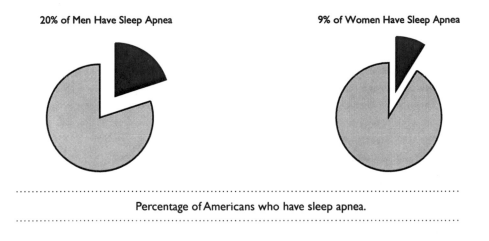

20% of Men Have Sleep Apnea

9% of Women Have Sleep Apnea

Percentage of Americans who have sleep apnea.

After menopause, sleep apnea in women is three times more common than before menopause (4).

A disturbing study of a group of truckers showed that 87 percent had some sign of sleep apnea (4). Since people with untreated sleep apnea have 15 times the normal risk of falling asleep at the wheel, truckers with sleep apnea pose a worrisome risk of major accidents. In fact, when a trucker dies in an accident, an average of 4.3 other victims die in that same accident.

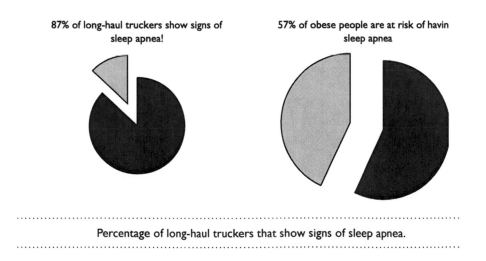

87% of long-haul truckers show signs of sleep apnea!

57% of obese people are at risk of havin sleep apnea

Percentage of long-haul truckers that show signs of sleep apnea.

Sleep Apnea Can Sneak Up On You

Untreated sleep apnea can be progressive, worsening over the course of 10 or 20 years without you realizing that you have it, until it may present a real threat to life.

On the Wednesday before Christmas of 1985, Reverend Allen felt himself slipping toward death. This 67-year-old retired minister had seen one doctor after another, searching for the reason for his declining health. Specialists had treated him for heart problems and a variety of other symptoms. But no one had been able to explain what was causing his problems. By December 1985, Reverend Allen was so weak he could hardly walk across his living room.

Now his only prayer was that he might make it through Christmas.

Reverend Allen had lacked energy all his life; even a little exertion wore him out. He slept poorly and never awakened refreshed. When he retired from preaching, he had looked forward to getting plenty of rest and finally feeling better. Instead he had felt more exhausted than ever. His health had become much worse.

He began to lose his coordination. Simple things, such as walking and writing, became difficult. His memory was failing and he would forget familiar words. This embarrassed and saddened him, for he had been a skilled craftsman with words, a preacher's most powerful tools. But now those tools seemed scattered and lost. Even his sense of humor had disappeared. The previous summer his wife had noticed a story in an insurance company magazine about a disorder called sleep apnea. The symptoms had rung a familiar bell— heavy snoring, daytime sleepiness, and exhaustion. She had awakened Reverend Allen, who was asleep as usual in his easy chair, and suggested that he might find the article interesting.

Indeed he did! The article described his symptoms exactly. Excited and hopeful, Reverend Allen took the article to his doctor. But his doctor was not particularly interested.

The next 6 months became a race with time as Reverend Allen's health rapidly deteriorated. His wife doggedly pursued their only lead— sleep apnea— through a long string of discouraging phone calls. Finally, they were put in touch with a new sleep disorders center in a nearby city. They made an appointment for an interview on the Wednesday before Christmas.

On the appointment day, Reverend Allen seemed so frail that his wife was afraid he might die on the way to the sleep center. She nearly canceled the appointment. But Reverend Allen was determined to try to make it through Christmas. "What's the difference," he had shrugged, "whether you go to Heaven from home or from the freeway?"

The sleep specialist immediately suspected severe sleep apnea. He rearranged his schedule so that Reverend Allen could have a sleep test the very next night. The doctor knew that if he delayed, he would be sorry for a very long time.

Sleep tests revealed that Reverend Allen had severe obstructive sleep apnea. He was immediately started on treatment with continuous positive airway pressure (CPAP) a breathing device that is used during sleep (see Chapter 10).

"And that," says Reverend Allen, "was a new beginning! The first morning after I went on CPAP, I woke up feeling refreshed. I wanted to take a walk!"

Three months later, this man, who had been near death, barely able to shuffle across his living room, was walking three-quarters of a mile every day. And, to his friends' delight and his own, his sense of humor had returned.

Reverend Allen's heart problems probably were the result of a lifetime of untreated sleep apnea. Treatment of sleep apnea can prevent, or even reverse, these medical problems. The sooner treatment is begun, the better the results.

Reverend Allen's story is dramatic. Not every case of long-term sleep apnea is so severe, and not every recovery is so striking. But in many ways, his story is typical—the snoring, the sleepiness, the fatigue, the loss of vigor, the threatening progress of an unidentified disease, the frustrations of seeking help where none seems available.

Most sleep apnea sufferers have followed a similar path. Today, more than 15 years after publication of the first edition of this book, the public and the medical community are becoming more aware of the signs, symptoms, and seriousness of sleep apnea. In addition, sleep specialists have learned more about the diagnosis and treatment of sleep apnea and other forms of sleep-disordered breathing.

As knowledge and awareness increase, and as more accredited sleep disorders centers are available, one must hope that people are more likely to be diagnosed at an earlier stage and can begin treatment before they develop severe medical complications.

The Top 10 Symptoms of Sleep Apnea

You may be the last person to know you have sleep apnea. After all, you are asleep when the problem occurs and it goes away when you wake up. Often, it is a friend or loved one who notices that someone's sleep and breathing during sleep are not quite normal.

So usually husbands, wives, children, and friends are the first to identify the top 10 most common symptoms of sleep apnea and sleep-disordered breathing. (You can read more about each of these symptoms in later chapters.)

Loud, Irregular Snoring, Snorts, Gasps, and Other Unusual Breathing Sounds During Sleep

Anyone who snores loudly and/or often is a sleep apnea suspect. The snoring stops when the person stops breathing and begins again, sometimes with a snort or a gasp, when the person takes the next breath.

Irregular snoring, with breathing that stops, is different from the quiet, relaxed sawing of ZZZs that most of us do occasionally, especially if we're sleeping on our back. Apnea-type snoring can be noisy, labored, and sometimes explosive. It may sound as though the person is struggling to breathe—which they are.

Another characteristic of severe apnea-type snoring is that it can happen in almost any position. Rolling over on the side often does not help, although some patients snore and have apnea only when sleeping on their back.

Heavy or labored breathing, without snoring, can be a sign of sleep-disordered breathing that is a close relative of sleep apnea and also needs medical attention.

Unfortunately, a person cannot count on the presence or absence of loud snoring alone to identify sleep apnea. A person may have sleep apnea even if the snoring is quiet or infrequent. The absence of snoring does not rule out sleep apnea as a diagnosis.

Finally, someone who sleeps alone may have sleep apnea without suspecting it at all. They will need to rely on the other nine signs of sleep apnea to suggest a visit with a sleep specialist.

Pauses in Breathing During Sleep

Everyone's breathing is irregular at certain times during sleep. Your breathing may pause for a moment just as you fall asleep or as you awaken, and breathing during dreams tends to speed up and slow down in an irregular manner. These are all normal changes in breathing while asleep.

However, a person with sleep apnea frequently stops breathing entirely, and may hold his or her breath for a surprisingly long time. Each of these periods during which breathing has stopped is called an apnea episode or an apnea event. An apnea event may last from 10 seconds to more than a minute.

Sleep specialists measure sleep apnea in several ways. One is the *Apnea Index,* which is the number of apnea events during an hour of sleep. Another measure is how long the apnea episodes last. If a person has an Apnea Index of 20 (20 apnea episodes per hour of sleep) and if the apnea episodes last more than 10 seconds, a sleep specialist would diagnose the person as having moderately severe sleep apnea.

Another measure of sleep apnea is the amount of oxygen in the blood, called *oxygen saturation*. If you are not breathing, you are not taking in oxygen, so the oxygen in the blood stream is gradually used up and the organs in the body are not receiving the oxygen they need. The brain is very sensitive to being deprived of oxygen.

By morning, a person with sleep apnea may have experienced hundreds of fairly long episodes of not breathing. Wouldn't that person be aware of such a struggle to breathe? No. People with sleep apnea have been deprived of decent sleep for a long time. They usually are so desperately sleep deprived that they barely awaken to breathe and seldom are aware of doing so. Occasionally, apnea patients will notice awakening briefly with a snort, particularly during naps or when they nod off in a sitting position. They are likely to describe their problem as "insomnia."

But most people with sleep apnea are the last to know it. Many have absolutely no complaints about their sleep. They will say they sleep "just fine," and only wish their bedmate would stop bothering them about their snoring.

But listen! A bed partner who says you stop breathing during sleep is probably not making it up! A tape recording of a person's sleeping sounds can be useful for convincing both that person and their doctor that he suffers from a breathing disorder during sleep.

Excessive Daytime Sleepiness

The most common sleep complaint of people with sleep apnea is that they get "too much sleep." Sleep specialists call this symptom *excessive daytime sleepiness* (EDS).

Two-thirds of sleep apnea patients suffer from some degree of EDS, and they may not even know it. They have lived with the effects of sleep apnea for so long, or it has crept up on them so gradually, that they do not know what "normal" feels like. They may think that they feel normal, that drowsiness is just a sign of getting older, or that maybe they just need a vacation.

The person with sleep apnea can think of endless explanations for why they fall asleep at their desk at work, at the wheel while driving, at the dinner table, after dinner on the sofa, at parties, at sporting events, and so on.

However, it is not normal to have to fight to stay awake, even in really boring meetings. If you *ever* are struggling against sleepiness during the day, you need to find out why, because that much drowsiness is not normal. Find out now before it further undermines your life.

Excessive daytime sleepiness results mainly from poor nighttime sleep—sleep that is interrupted over and over throughout the night by repeated apnea events. Someone with sleep apnea does not get enough sleep, and that sleep is of poor quality. As a result, people with sleep apnea build up a *sleep debt*—an ongoing need for sleep that carries over into their daytime life. Their sleep debt pressures them to fall asleep easily and frequently during the daytime—at their desk at work, while reading or watching TV, and while driving (see illustration on page 17) (1).

Unexplained Fatigue

Fatigue is another common problem for people with sleep apnea. Fatigue is different from sleepiness. Rather than a desire to go to sleep, fatigue is a sense of feeling exhausted, drained. People with sleep apnea typically feel fatigued much of the time. Often, because their apnea has been present for years and has gotten progressively worse, they are not even aware that they are more tired than normal. Or they assume that their fatigue is simply a normal sign of aging.

Again, as with drowsiness, a constant feeling of exhaustion is *not normal*. Exhaustion is not an inevitable sign of age. A person feeling fatigued much of the time probably has a medical problem. It may or may not be sleep apnea. But a physician should certainly consider sleep apnea as a possible cause of unexplained fatigue, and refer a chronically fatigued patient to a sleep clinic for testing.

CASE STUDY

Mr. Bell's wife pleaded with him to see a doctor about his gasping and irregular breathing during sleep. But Mr. Bell was in excellent physical condition, and at the age of 46 could outrun much younger men in 10- kilometer races. He had seen a TV show about sleep problems and knew that some apnea and snoring can be normal, so he ignored his wife's request.

A life insurance company reviewed Mr. Bell's medical records and noticed that the doctor's note suggested "possible sleep apnea," so they denied him insurance. Mr. Bell went to a sleep center, hoping to prove he was in perfect health. Instead he learned that, in fact, he had moderately severe apnea.

Mr. Bell received treatment for his sleep apnea, and a follow-up study of his sleep showed an excellent response. His insurance application was approved, which pleased him; in addition, Mr. Bell realized that he felt much better. He was amazed that he had not noticed the signs of sleep apnea before treatment.

The moral of Mr. Bell's story is clear: if your bedmate thinks you have sleep apnea, he is probably right, even if you don't feel ill. Some people can tolerate very significant amounts of sleep apnea without being aware of it. Apparently, they do not notice a deterioration in the quality of their sleep or their daytime alertness, nor are they bothered by "insomnia" or fatigue. Mr. Bell is typical of former sleep apnea patients after treatment—they are astonished at feeling so much more wide-awake, energetic, and alive!

Obesity

And more than half of obese people have sleep apnea, and don't know it.

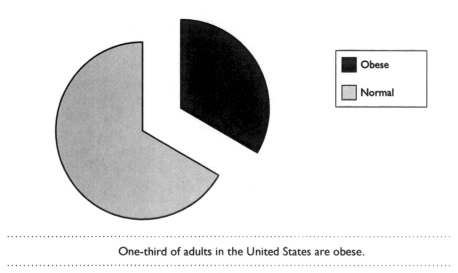

One-third of adults in the United States are obese.

A complicated relationship exists between weight and sleep apnea: sleep apnea makes the weight problem worse, and vice versa. Often, late-onset diabetes (also called type II diabetes) appears when adults become overweight, and these three factors—obesity, diabetes, and sleep apnea—working together can further worsen cardiovascular and heart diseases (see illustration at the top of page 9).

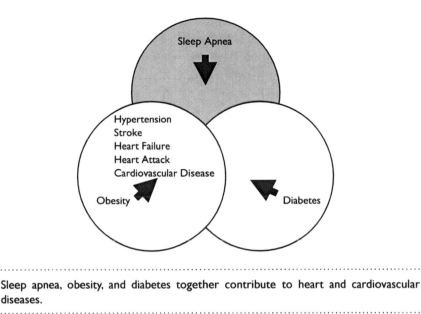

Sleep apnea, obesity, and diabetes together contribute to heart and cardiovascular diseases.

Losing weight usually helps the sleep apnea, but most people cannot lose weight until after the sleep apnea has been treated. The sleep apnea-obesity relationship is described in more detail in Chapter 11.

Not everyone who is overweight suffers from sleep apnea, nor is everyone who has sleep apnea necessarily overweight. In fact, individuals who are quite thin can have severe sleep apnea.

CASE STUDY

Mr. Johnson was a 29-year-old man who snored badly and had been tired "for years." His wife had noticed pauses in his breathing during sleep, but they were infrequent, and she was a good sleeper so she didn't mind his snoring.

Several doctors over several years had performed thorough medical examinations and had concluded that stress or underlying depression was the likely cause of Mr. Johnson's chronic tiredness. During his last evaluation, he mentioned the snoring and the apnea that his wife had observed, but he was told he was "too young and too thin" to have any trouble with sleep apnea. Mr. Johnson eventually was studied in a sleep center, and it was discovered that he stopped breathing 43 times an hour. With treatment using nasal CPAP (see Chapter 10), Mr. Johnson's fatigue disappeared entirely.

Changes in Alertness or Memory

Over the years, people with untreated sleep apnea may experience a loss of alertness, and difficulty concentrating, which can contribute to auto accidents and job difficulties. Memory loss is common in sleep apnea, and may be blamed on "just getting older." However, once the sleep apnea has been effectively treated, many of these faculties may return, proving that "getting older" was not the culprit.

Changes in Mood, Personality, or Behavior

Sleep apnea can mimic depression, laziness, or personality change. Increased irritability, shortness of temper, or "crabbiness" are very often caused by sleep apnea but, like excessive daytime sleepiness, can be explained away as the result of, for example, stress, job dissatisfaction, or relationship problems.

Family and friends often are the first to notice behavioral signs of sleep apnea: a gradual shift in sleeping or napping habits, a decline in the person's energy level, reduced productivity at home or at work, or changes in mood or disposition. Any of these changes in behavior, which the affected person might not notice, may suggest sleep apnea.

CASE STUDY

M r. Arnold was under a lot of stress. His business was in trouble from new competition. His wife was drinking heavily, and their marriage seemed to be breaking down. His business partner was concerned that he was gaining weight, seemed irritable and depressed, and was not his usual outgoing self with the office staff and customers. Mr. Arnold was distracted in business meetings, and his once photographic memory for business statistics was slipping badly.

His partner suggested that he see a psychologist and get help to deal with his stress, depression, and marital problems. He took his partner's advice. But counseling did not help, and his family doctor referred him to a psychiatrist. The psychiatrist noted his snoring and sleepiness and sent him for testing at a sleep center, where he was found to be suffering from sleep apnea. Treatment resolved his personality change, memory problems, and poor work performance.

Unexplained changes in mental sharpness or in personality should arouse a suspicion of possible sleep apnea if they are accompanied by apnea during sleep, fatigue, weight gain, or other symptoms mentioned in this chapter.

Impotence, Morning Headaches, and Bed-wetting

Impotence, morning headaches, and bed-wetting are other symptoms sometimes associated with sleep apnea. Few people have all 10 symptoms. Most people show only one or two obvious signs of the disorder.

It is important to emphasize that any of the symptoms of sleep apnea might also be caused by other, possibly harmful, conditions. For this and other reasons, a person who suspects sleep apnea or any other type of sleep-disordered breathing should talk with a specialist in sleep disorders medicine, so that other disorders can be ruled out and the correct diagnosis made.

◆ Summary

A person shows signs of sleep apnea syndrome that may affect his health:

✓ If the person stops breathing for more than 10 seconds at a time.
✓ If this happens more than five times during an hour of sleep.

The following are the most common signs and symptoms of sleep apnea:

1. Loud, irregular snoring
2. Snorts, gasps, and other unusual breathing sounds during sleep
3. Long pauses in breathing during sleep
4. Excessive daytime sleepiness
5. Fatigue
6. Obesity
7. Changes in alertness, memory, personality, or behavior
8. Impotence
9. Morning headaches
10. Bed-wetting

If you have loud, irregular snoring or labored breathing during sleep plus any of the other preceding symptoms, you should ask your doctor to refer you to an accredited sleep center for evaluation.

Sleep Apnea Is Hard on Your Heart

Untreated sleep apnea can cause:

- Twenty-three times higher risk of heart attack.
- Ten times higher risk of stroke.
- More than two times higher risk of heart failure.
- Hypertension: the more severe the sleep apnea, the more severe the hypertension.

Untreated sleep apnea is as harmful to your heart as:

- Smoking
- Diabetes
- Obesity

Sleep Apnea Causes Heart and Lung Problems

Sleep apnea is hard on the heart. Untreated, sleep apnea can cause irregular heart rhythms, enlargement of the heart, heart attacks, heart failure, high blood pressure, and strokes, and it contributes to other aspects of cardiovascular disease (see illustration at the top of page 13) (1).

Strokes are three times more common in heavy snorers than in nonsnorers (2) and 10 times more common in people with sleep apnea (2,3). Heart attack is more than 20 times more likely in people with untreated sleep apnea (3). Middle-aged people with untreated sleep apnea have a 35% greater risk of heart disease than healthy people.

The cardiovascular effects of untreated sleep apnea result in the nocturnal sudden death of approximately 2,000 to 3,000 people per year in the United States (4).

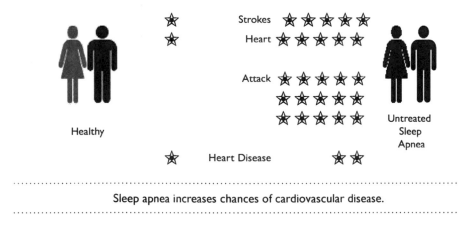

Sleep apnea increases chances of cardiovascular disease.

Let's look at some of the nuts and bolts of how sleep apnea damages people's health.

Struggle, Panic, and Suffocation

Sleep apnea makes the heart and lungs struggle to do their job. With each episode of apnea, the act of snoring sucks the pressure down in the chest cavity, and the heart has to pump harder to make up for this abnormal pressure difference.

In addition, with each apnea event, there is a brief awakening, so short that you wouldn't notice it, but it causes a surge in epinephrine (adrenalin) (the "fight-or-flight" response), which charges up the sympathetic nervous system and increases blood pressure. This happens many times during the night, and it has harmful effects upon the heart as well as other organs.

Over a period of years, these effects can become life-threatening.

Low Blood Oxygen Concentration

Each apnea event reduces the amount of air reaching the lungs, the blood stream, and the brain. The brain is particularly susceptible to low oxygen. A shortage of oxygen during the night is typical in a person with sleep apnea, and causes much of the long-term harm resulting from sleep apnea. If the low blood oxygen is severe and continues over a long period, it can unfavorably affect the brain. This may explain the changes in personality, memory, alertness, decision-making ability, and coordination seen in people with sleep apnea (5).

High Blood Pressure

High blood pressure is one important cardiovascular effect of both low blood oxygen and the "fight-or-flight" response. High blood pressure is seen in 35 to 50 percent of sleep apnea patients (see illustration at the top of page 14). The more severe the sleep apnea, the higher the blood pressure elevation (6,7).

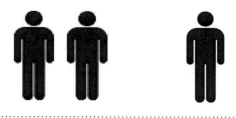

One of every three men with high blood pressure has sleep apnea.

Chronic high blood pressure results in enlargement of the heart, which is a risk factor for stroke and heart failure (8). Sleep apnea also causes changes in the walls of arteries, in the nervous system, and in the flow of hormones that regulate many organs in the body.

Blood pressure may be indirectly improved when the treatment of sleep apnea allows the patient to lose weight and enjoy regular exercise. Excess weight contributes to high blood pressure, and regular exercise can help to lower blood pressure.

Patients on high doses of blood pressure medications should make sure their doctors follow them carefully after their sleep apnea is treated to see if they need less medication. Sometimes symptoms of low blood pressure may develop, because their bodies no longer require as much medication.

Sleep apnea contributes notably to a particular type of high blood pressure: unusually high pressure in the artery that carries blood from the right side of the heart to the lungs. This occurs mainly in people who have other health problems and already have low blood oxygen when they are awake. In time, this condition can lead to enlargement of the right side of the heart and fluid congestion in the lungs (8–11).

Arrhythmia

Arrhythmia (abnormal heart rhythm) is seen in more than 90 percent of sleep apnea patients (see illustration at the top of page 15) (11). Abnormal slowing of the heart, long pauses (more than 2 seconds), extra beats, and several other types of arrhythmias are associated with sleep apnea. People with sleep apnea may have a higher than normal risk of sudden death from heart failure during the night, probably because of a fatal arrhythmia (12).

The work of the lungs is affected by changes in blood pressure (described earlier) that result from low blood oxygen. In addition, the low oxygen and high carbon dioxide concentrations in the blood result in abnormal blood chemistry. These changes in blood chemistry also disturb the functioning of the lungs (13,14).

The combined damage from cardiopulmonary disturbances—abnormal blood pressure relationships in the heart and lungs, repeated bouts of "fight-or-flight," abnormal blood chemistry from too much carbon dioxide and too little oxygen, arrhythmias—is thought by most sleep specialists to be the greatest long-term danger to health from sleep apnea1 (see illustration on page 15) (15).

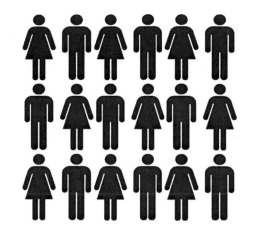

Abnormal Heart Rhythm

Normal
Heart Rhythm

Nine of 10 people with sleep apnea have abnormal heart rhythmias.

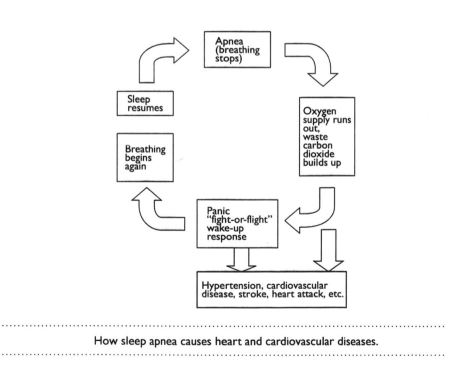

How sleep apnea causes heart and cardiovascular diseases.

Treatment of Sleep Apnea Lowers Cardiovascular Risks

After people receive effective treatment for their sleep apnea, their risks of cardiovascular disease decrease significantly (see illustration at the top of page 16).

Some people's hypertension improves so much that they no longer need blood pressure medication. Irregular heart rhythms and heart failure may improve, and the chances of dying from cardiovascular disease return to nearly normal (15–17).

As shown in the following illustration, a person with severe untreated sleep apnea has three times the normal risk of death from cardiovascular disease.

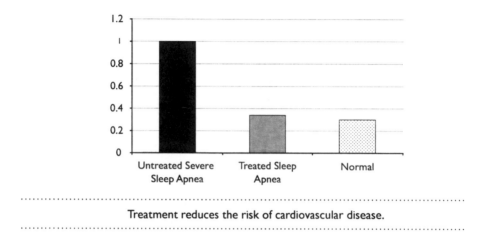

Treatment reduces the risk of cardiovascular disease.

In the following illustration, you can see that once sleep apnea has been treated, the risk of death from cardiovascular disease decreases to near normal.

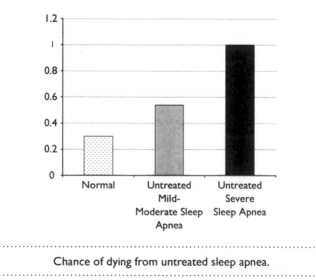

Chance of dying from untreated sleep apnea.

Treatment of sleep apnea can also restore vitality and energy level and improve the person's mood and outlook, so that they are awake, alert, and able to enjoy life more than they have for many years.

Driving Sleepy: Sleep Apnea Causes Auto Crashes

Sleepy Drivers Are as Dangerous as Drunk Drivers

People with severe, untreated sleep apnea have a *15-fold greater risk* of an automobile wreck than normal people (1).

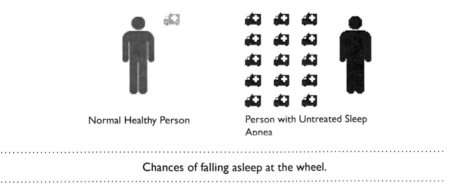

Normal Healthy Person

Person with Untreated Sleep Apnea

Chances of falling asleep at the wheel.

The National Sleep Foundation estimates that 200,000 sleep-related motor vehicle crashes occur every year, and that includes 2,700 fatalities. In 1996, the American Medical Association urged all physicians to learn about sleep disorders and to warn their patients of the dangers of driving and working while fatigued or sleepy (2).

One in five sleep apnea patients admit to having had auto accidents from falling asleep at the wheel (3). People who have had a near miss from dozing off while driving are at *very* high risk of having a serious crash.

The hazard of automobile accidents from untreated sleep apnea is very similar to the hazard from alcohol (4). Research has shown that, like a drunk driver, a sleepy driver tends to underestimate his or her degree of impairment, not only the ability to stay awake but also to perform divided-attention tasks such as observing the surroundings, staying in the correct lane, adjusting speed and position, and anticipating other drivers' behavior (5).

Sleepiness while driving can develop gradually over weeks or months. Before having an actual automobile accident, most apnea patients have had very brief "microsleeps" while driving. They nod off for an instant, maybe with a prolonged eye blink or a head bob. A 2-second microsleep is equal to driving 200 feet while sound asleep—plenty of time to hit a tree or to cross into oncoming traffic and cause a death that will never be forgotten (4). Auto accidents among people with sleep apnea are so common that some sleep clinics give each sleep apnea patient a letter advising him not to drive until he has received treatment.

The sleepy driver may ignore or not admit the warning signals of a potentially life-threatening episode of sleepiness. The family of a person with life-threatening sleepiness may have observed him or her repeatedly falling asleep, even on short trips; yet the driver may absolutely deny that she is sleepy or dangerous.

The failure to appreciate this danger may come from lack of awareness, pride, or denial of the problem. One study compared the accident records between men and women with untreated sleep apnea. Men were about four times more likely than women to drive while sleepy and to have automobile accidents (6). Refusing to be a passenger might inspire the sleepy driver to acknowledge the danger.

Transportation Workers Are a Special Risk Group

In the transportation industry and in the workplace, untreated sleep apnea is a public danger. Imagine drowsy school bus drivers, commercial airline and steamship pilots, railroad engineers, truck drivers, heavy equipment operators, and carpool drivers. There are flagrant examples of drowsiness-based disasters in each of these fields. People in these occupations who *ever* experience drowsiness on the job have an obligation either to identify and treat the cause of their drowsiness or to change occupations.

Studies of long-haul truck drivers have found that nearly half of them have obvious signs suggesting sleep apnea (7). When truckers were actually tested for sleep apnea in the sleep lab, the results showed that 17% had mild sleep apnea, 6% had moderate sleep apnea, and 5% had severe sleep apnea (see chart on page 19) (8), and all of these were untreated and still on the highway.

A 2006 task force of occupational medicine and sleep disorders experts recommended that every 2 years, when commercial drivers must renew their licenses, the commercial driver medical examiners evaluate every driver for fitness to drive based on drowsiness or other symptoms suggesting an untreated sleep disorder. These symptoms would include snoring, excessive daytime sleepiness, stopping breathing during sleep, obesity, or hypertension. The medical examiner could require the driver to have a sleep study, undergo treatment, and show certification from a sleep specialist that treatment is effective (5).

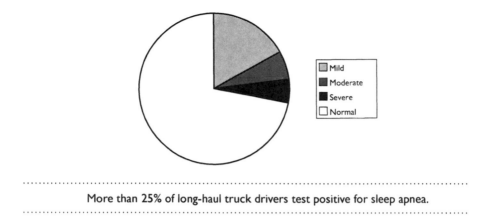

More than 25% of long-haul truck drivers test positive for sleep apnea.

Effectiveness of Treatment Must Be Verified

Once treatment for sleep apnea has begun, it is important for both health and safety to make sure that the treatment is actually having an effect. Feeling cured is not the same as being cured, as the following case illustrates.

CASE STUDY

Mr. Rodgers was diagnosed with moderately severe obstructive sleep apnea and underwent UPPP (uvulopalatopharyngoplasty) surgery (discussed in Chapter 7). His snoring disappeared, he felt better, and he no longer fell asleep at the wrong times. The surgeon recommended that he return to the sleep center for a retest to see how much improvement had actually been achieved by the surgery. Mr. Rodgers refused to be retested because he was "absolutely sure" he was cured.

Six months later, Mr. Rodgers fell asleep while driving and wrecked his car. In retrospect, he could recall occasionally feeling drowsy even though he had improved significantly after surgery. A follow-up sleep study showed that he still had 50 percent of his sleep apnea. Further treatment resulted in full control of his symptoms.

If you suffer from excessive drowsiness, you owe it to yourself, your family, your coworkers, and others on the highway to refrain from driving until you have been tested to determine the cause of your problem and have begun effective treatment.

Hangover from Sleeping Pills

Another cause of sleepy-driver crashes is the morning hangover effect from a sleeping pill taken the night before. People with sleep problems—including some with sleep apnea—may take sleeping pills in an effort to improve their sleep. The risk of having an automobile crash or a workplace accident is very high if a person attempts to drive before a sedative has completely worn off.

Older sleep medications, particularly the benzodiazepines (lorazepam [Ativan], triazplam [Halcion], temazepam [Restoril], and others) are noted for undesirable side effects, including next-day drowsiness. Their side effects prompted the search for more tolerable sleep medications.

The new generation of nonbenzodiazepine sleep medications (for example, zolpidem [Ambien], eszopiclone [Lunesta], and zaleplon [Sonata]) are faster-acting, short-lasting sleeping medications with fewer side effects. Nevertheless, after numerous tragic morning-after crashes, these sleep medications now carry a warning label about the danger of sedation the following day.

Thus, even the "short-acting" sleep medications should be used with great care. Some people are more susceptible than others to the hangover effects of sleep medications. This is especially the case in a person with untreated sleep apnea who already suffers from chronic daytime drowsiness.

Morning drowsiness should be regarded as a serious potential side effect of sleep medications, and the presence of alcohol may intensify the effects.

Sleep Apnea Invades Health, Home, and Workplace

Sleep apnea is linked with medical problems:

- Frequent automobile and workplace accidents
- Five times greater risk of stroke
- Twenty times greater risk of heart attack
- Irregular heart rhythms
- Heart failure
- High blood pressure
- Diabetes

Sleep apnea also causes family, workplace, and mental problems:

- Daytime sleepiness
- Poor memory and decision making
- Job problems
- Poor coordination
- Depression
- Irritability
- Mood swings
- Isolation from friends and family

People with sleep apnea pay a high price over the years. Their health, family life, and career really suffer from the poor quality of their sleep, from their nightly struggle to breathe, and from the low oxygen supply in their blood during the night. Family, friends, employers, and business associates of people with untreated sleep apnea also pay a high price because of negative changes in personality, decreased work performance, and overall diminished ability to fulfill their social and emotional responsibilities.

Sleep Apnea Sabotages Family and Career

Social and Psychological Effects

The fatigue and sleepiness caused by sleep apnea can literally destroy a person's life and pull a family apart. Poor quality of sleep coupled with nighttime low oxygen levels can cause actual damage to the nervous system. Climbers on Mt. Everest know that the lack of oxygen at high elevation causes difficulty thinking clearly. People with sleep apnea may take in even less oxygen than they would at the summit of Mt. Everest (1).

Work performance can be profoundly undermined. Absenteeism can be a problem for people with sleep apnea. They tend to miss work more frequently, arrive at work late, and become drowsy or fall asleep on the job, so that even when they are at their desk, they really are not there.

Sleep apnea causes a decline in the ability to think clearly. People with sleep apnea score lower than normal on tests for attention and concentration and on other tests of brain activity (2). Where once they were sharp and on top of their job, they now have difficulty making decisions, evaluating information, concentrating, planning, organizing, and carrying out plans. Sleep apnea leads to memory loss, mental disorganization, poor judgment, rigid thinking, and difficulty staying motivated (3). Not surprisingly, employers of people affected by sleep apnea may notice a decline in job performance. Bosses and colleagues seldom understand the problem and often assume that the employee's behavior is due to drugs, alcohol, or serious personality problems. Promotions are missed, jobs are lost, and promising careers are sidetracked.

Home life and social life also suffer. People with severe untreated sleep apnea simply become unable to function in the normal, everyday world.

People with sleep apnea tend to become socially isolated and alienated from their partners and children. The fatigue and sleepiness of the sleep apnea sufferer lead him or her to participate less and less in family activities and relationships and to spend more and more time withdrawn or sleeping. Family life often begins to feel more like a burden than a source of support (4). The family may become critical of his inactivity, decreased work around the house, or negative and crabby attitude. The result is a puzzled, resentful, increasingly uncommunicative family. These problems may contribute to marital conflicts, child-raising difficulties, and divorce.

Psychological problems and mood changes are frequent results of sleep apnea. Irritability is common in people with moderate to severe sleep apnea, as are other personality changes, such as depression, memory impairment, confusion, anger, and even physical abuse.

The loss of mental acuity usually is so gradual that the person may not realize it is happening. First he may find that reading is a chore, so he will read less. Then he may have trouble concentrating on other tasks or remembering words. It may not be until after his sleep apnea is under treatment and his mental facility begins to return that he realizes how much he has lost.

To summarize, driving accidents may be the most immediate threat of death from sleep apnea. In the longer term, sleep apnea leads to life-threatening medical complications and psychological and social difficulties. Most of these consequences can be lessened or eliminated with treatment of the apnea. Treatment is discussed in Chapter 10.

Diagnosing and Treating Sleep Apnea

Anyone can develop sleep apnea, even you!

- One of every four middle-aged men
- One of every 10 middle-aged women
- Even children

Sleep apnea has been around forever, but only recently recognized.
Many doctors are not accustomed to looking for signs of sleep apnea.
Treating sleep apnea can lower your risk of serious medical problems.

- Heart disease
- High blood pressure
- Diabetes
- Automobile crashes

Visit a sleep specialist to find out if you have sleep apnea or another condition that needs treatment.

Who Suffers from Sleep Apnea?

When does a person's tendency toward sleep apnea first arise? This is difficult to pinpoint because sleep apnea results from the combination of several risk factors.

Sleep apnea can be found at all ages. In some people, the tendency may be present at birth. Sleep apnea may be the later stage of a breathing disorder that begins early in life as a slight breathing abnormality—some part of the automatic breathing reflex that is slightly irregular.

A breathing abnormality is more likely to develop into sleep apnea when other important risk factors are present:

- Obesity
- An insensitive breathing reflex (see Chapter 6)
- A slight failure in coordination between the breathing muscles
- An upper airway that is narrowed or obstructed by blockages, for example, in the nasal passages, large tonsils or adenoids, a large tongue, or a short lower jaw

Any of these factors may combine, so that a slight breathing instability in a young person gradually can evolve into a permanent abnormality in sleep breathing in an adult (1).

Some tendencies to develop sleep apnea probably are inherited. For example, a person may inherit an airway whose shape is easily obstructed. Or he may inherit a weak breathing response to carbon dioxide. Either one or a combination of several inherited factors may set the stage for a person to develop sleep apnea (2).

Gender is a factor in the development of sleep apnea. Men are about three times more likely to have sleep apnea than women (3). The reasons for this difference may have to do with sexual differences in the structure of the airway or in muscle tone. The effects of sex hormones may also be a factor (for example, progesterone in women versus testosterone in men).

Extra body weight is another factor. Obese people suffer a much higher incidence of sleep apnea than people of ideal weight (see Chapter 11).

In terms of age, sleep apnea is primarily a condition of middle age or older. This is true for several reasons. First, with age there is a loss of muscle tone in the throat during sleep. Second, when people do have untreated sleep apnea, the condition becomes worse as they grow older. Third, body weight tends to increase with age, often beginning after age 40. By the time the symptoms of sleep apnea are serious enough to attract medical attention, the person may be in his or her 40s or 50s and may be suffering from obesity, pulmonary complications, arrhythmia, or even congestive heart failure. The average age of patients in one sleep clinic was reported to be 52.4 years.

However, sleep apnea can occur at any age. Children can have sleep apnea. In fact, now that obesity affects one-third of US children, and tonsillectomies are less common than they used to be, sleep apnea is probably more prevalent in children than it was a generation ago. Children who have enlarged tonsils or adenoids or who are obese are the most likely to develop sleep apnea. (See Chapter 12 for information about apnea in infants and about sudden infant death syndrome [SIDS] and Chapter 13 for more about sleep apnea in older children.)

A number of drugs aggravate sleep apnea. These include alcohol, sedatives, hypnotic drugs (sleeping pills), and some heart medications (short-acting beta blockers, such as propranolol) (see the Appendix).

Why Haven't You Heard of Sleep Apnea Before?

It has been estimated that 20 million Americans may have sleep apnea (5). Among 30 to 60 year olds, 1 of every 4 men and 1 of every 10 women show some signs of sleep apnea. In a study of industrial workers in Israel, one of every five was classified as having some degree of sleep apnea (6). These are surprisingly large numbers of people, considering that a few years ago hardly anybody had ever heard of sleep apnea.

So if sleep apnea is this common, why haven't you heard about it before? The answer is that sleep apnea has always been around, but it was not recognized by the medical community until recently.

One of the earliest descriptions of sleep apnea was published in 1877 by an observant medical man named W. H. Broadbent. He did not call the condition sleep apnea, but he described the two major types of apnea that today are called obstructive apnea and central apnea.

During the late 1800s, several additional reports were published about patients who suffered from abnormal daytime sleepiness and had difficulty breathing while asleep. In 1890, an early American neurologist and toxicologist named Silas Weir Mitchell wrote the first detailed accounts of a breathing disorder that occurred during sleep and began to unravel the mystery of what causes sleep apnea.

Unfortunately for those suffering from sleep apnea, bacteria were soon after identified as the cause of certain diseases, and medical attention focused on sleep diseases that were caused by microbes, such as sleeping sickness, and little interest or credence was given to other kinds of sleep disorders or their causes. As a result, much of what had been learned or suggested about sleep disorders lapsed into neglect.

It was not until the 1950s that several groups of scientists began to make careful observations of actual sleeping people. They developed an electronic technique for measuring and studying sleep, called polysomnography (see Chapter 6). Using this technique, they began to discover interesting things about what goes on during sleep. They learned, for example, that sleep is not at all a time of peaceful inactivity. This unexpected discovery stimulated an explosion of interest in sleep research and intensified the quest for a better understanding of sleep, both normal and abnormal.

It soon became apparent that events during sleep can profoundly affect a person's health. As explained by Dr. William Dement, one of the leaders in this field, "It is possible for individuals to be entirely normal awake and deathly ill asleep" (7). Thus, a new field of medicine—sleep disorders medicine—began to take shape.

In the past 15 years, sleep researchers have learned how to recognize the signs of various abnormal sleep conditions—sleep apnea and other forms of sleep-disordered breathing, narcolepsy, nocturnal myoclonus, idiopathic central nervous system hypersomnolence, and others—that previously had been difficult or impossible to diagnose. Physicians are becoming better informed and are beginning to diagnose sleep apnea in patients who previously might simply have been treated for insomnia, heart problems, or some other symptom.

Confirming the Diagnosis and Treating Sleep Apnea

Once you have been given a tentative diagnosis of sleep apnea or a similar sleep/breathing disorder, an all-night sleep test should be arranged. Proper testing is important both to confirm the presence of a sleep disorder and to distinguish one sleep disorder from another. An incorrect diagnosis, leading to incorrect treatment, can be a serious error. For example, medications prescribed for narcolepsy or insomnia can actually worsen sleep apnea, so a correct diagnosis is very important.

Other Sleep Disorders Can Have Similar Symptoms

Narcolepsy is a sleep disorder in which people have irresistible "sleep attacks" at inappropriate times, somewhat as in sleep apnea. However, narcolepsy is a distinct neurological disorder with its own characteristic symptoms (cataplexy, sleep paralysis, and hypnagogic hallucinations) not found in sleep apnea.

Insomnia is sometimes confused with sleep apnea. Insomnia has numerous causes, and only a few people who have insomnia also have sleep apnea.

Two other sleep disorders sometimes occur alone or along with sleep apnea. These are *periodic limb movement in sleep* (PLMS, also called periodic leg movement disorder, PLMD, or nocturnal myoclonus) and *restless leg syndrome* (RLS). Both of these can cause daytime sleepiness, but, appropriate testing by an experienced sleep disorders specialist will avoid confusing one sleep disorder with another.

An overnight sleep test will:

Confirm whether you actually have sleep apnea or another form of sleep-disordered breathing

Determine the type of sleep/breathing disorder, which must be known in order to select the appropriate treatment

Rule out other sleep disorders

Chapters 6 through 10 of this book will take you through the processes of diagnosis and treatment of sleep apnea. Chapter 6 describes the three types of sleep apnea. Chapter 8 discusses some of the difficulties in diagnosing sleep apnea. Testing for sleep apnea is described in Chapter 9. Treatment choices are discussed in Chapter 10.

Chapter 7 is included for those readers who would like a better understanding of sleep and the causes of sleep apnea.

◆ Summary

✓ Sleep apnea is not yet widely recognized by family doctors.

✓ Sleep apnea can occur at any age but is most common in middle age, particularly among men and obese people.

✓ Sleep apnea is treatable.

✓ Sleep apnea can devastate a person's career, wreak havoc on family and social life, and cause psychological and memory problems.

Sleep apnea can be life-threatening if not treated. It results in:

- Automobile accidents
- Workplace accidents
- Abnormal blood chemistry
- High blood pressure
- Arrhythmia (irregular heartbeat)
- Other heart complications
- Lung complications
- Loss of alertness, memory, concentration
- Death

Normal Sleep, Snoring, and Sleep Apnea

- Sleep apnea causes sleep deprivation and sleep debt by reducing:
  - The amount of sleep
  - The quality of sleep
- Sleep apnea is caused by one or both of the following:
  - Obstructions in the breathing passages (partial obstruction causes snoring)
  - Faulty nervous system and muscle control of breathing reflexes
- Snoring often leads to sleep apnea, which may become worse over the years.

This chapter is for the reader who likes to understand how things work. But anyone can understand the causes of sleep apnea, and that understanding will help make it seem less frightening or mysterious.

This chapter will also equip you to discuss treatment options with your doctor, play an active role in choosing the treatment, and carry through on treatment.

Sleep—Normal and Abnormal

To understand the causes and results of sleep apnea, it helps to know a little about what happens during a normal night's sleep.

Why Do We Sleep?

Nobody knows exactly why we sleep. At one time, people thought that sleep was just a rest period for our brains. Then polysomnography was developed. This technology allows scientists to make electrical recordings of brain activities during sleep. Scientists were surprised to discover that brains are anything but idle during sleep.

Some theories suggested that we sleep to overcome body fatigue. Our bodies do seem to overcome fatigue during sleep, but studies have shown that it is our brain, not our muscles, that requires sleep in order to feel rested and function normally.

How Much Sleep Do We Need?

The amount of sleep needed varies from person to person, and also depends on age and circumstances.

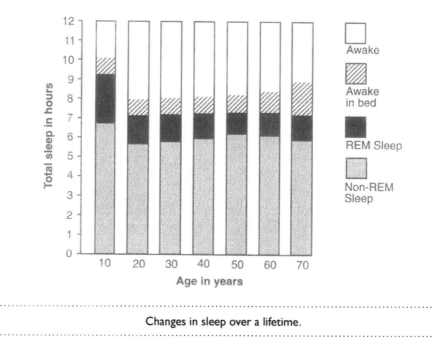

Changes in sleep over a lifetime.

It used to be said that babies needed 21 hours of sleep per day, but now we know that the need for sleep varies a great deal from infant to infant. Sixteen year olds seem to need approximately 10 or 11 hours of sleep, and this decreases to about 8 hours for an average adult. Occasional healthy, alert adults do fine on 4 hours of sleep, but that is rare. The record for habitually short sleep seems to be about 3 hours per night (1). No one has ever been documented to need no sleep.

What happens if people are experimentally deprived of sleep for several days? Sleep deprivation upsets the body's physiological systems: hormones, immune system, blood pressure regulation, digestive system, and urine production. Normally, many of our physiological processes have a 24-hour rhythm that cycles up and down. The acts of going to sleep and waking up in the morning send signals to our biological clock to keep those rhythms synchronized with each other. A person who is not sleeping well or whose sleep schedule is irregular (for example, because of shift work) does not send regular signals to reset his or her clock each day and keep the rhythms running smoothly. When the daily rhythms are not synchronized—as in someone working the night shift—the body shows signs of this disturbance. For example, people doing shift work have higher rates of digestive disorders, headaches, and some types of cancer.

In terms of behavior, sleep-deprived people have periodic bouts of drowsiness, as their built-in biological clock tries to make them go to sleep. Their ability to concentrate decreases, and their ability to think becomes dull. The effects of sleep deprivation on thinking and memory are especially damaging in school-aged children and teenagers, many of whom are seriously sleep deprived (2).

Sleep-deprived people also may become irritable and disoriented, and may have dreamlike hallucinations. Reactions become slow and erratic. This is why sleep-deprived drivers have more automobile accidents. Research shows that if a person sleeps for only 7 hours per night for a week, his reaction time will have slowed down enough to interfere with tasks such as driving. Nine hours of sleep are needed, consistently, every night, for one's reaction time to be at its best (3).

By itself, partial sleep deprivation is not fatal. However, it certainly causes fatalities when it interferes with the ability to perform normally on the highway or in the workplace. When a long-haul truck driver falls asleep at the wheel and crashes, an average of four more people die with him. Driving while sleepy is equivalent to driving drunk (4).

Sleep Quantity, Sleep Quality, and Sleep Debt

To be at our best, each of us needs a certain quantity of sleep every night. If we do not get enough sleep, we tend to build up a *sleep debt*. This leads to a tendency to feel drowsy during the day and to fall asleep more readily.

But the *quantity* of sleep we get is not the whole story. Equally important is the *quality* of our sleep. Does it come in nice, large, continuous blocks, or is it fragmented into short bits? Do we get enough "deep" sleep?

Sleep apnea causes repeated awakenings during the night. This decreases the quantity of sleep, and also reduces the quality of sleep by breaking up its structure and continuity. People with sleep apnea completely miss out on some of the normal and important stages of sleep.

Let's look a little more closely at what goes on in your brain while you are sleeping.

The Stages of Normal Sleep

The quality of sleep is related to the sequence of sleep stages that the brain passes through during the night.

After you go to sleep, the activities of your brain and body settle into a fairly predictable pattern. There are two kinds of sleep: REM (rapid eye movement) sleep and non-REM (or NREM) sleep. REM and NREM sleep alternate with each other during the night.

NREM sleep is *quiet* sleep. Your breathing and brain activity are slow and regular, and your body is quiet and relaxed. You may dream, but the dreams will be more thoughtlike than emotional.

REM sleep, in contrast, is *active* sleep. There are active changes in your physiology during REM sleep. For example, your breathing becomes irregular. You may stop breathing every now and then for several seconds. Your body temperature rises, and the blood circulation in your brain increases. The large muscles of your body—your leg and arm muscles—actually become paralyzed: you cannot move them except for little twitches of your face and fingertips. But your eye muscles become very active and move your eyes back and forth as if they were watching a ping-pong match. This, of course, is the rapid eye movement that led to the term *REM sleep*. Most, but not all, of your dreaming occurs during REM sleep. The most vivid, intense, emotional dreams almost always occur during REM sleep.

A typical night's sleep begins with quiet NREM sleep. During the first hour of sleep, NREM progress through four stages, from light to heavy sleep. Then, rather abruptly, about 70 to 90 minutes from the beginning of sleep, sleep lightens from its deepest level to reach the first REM period. That first REM sleep period usually lasts about 10 minutes. It ends when sleep shifts back into lighter stage 2 NREM sleep. Then sleep begins to deepen and the cycle starts all over again.

This cycle takes about 90 minutes and repeats itself throughout the night. Early in the night, the REM periods are shorter. During the second half of the night, REM periods become longer, sometimes as long as 60 minutes, separated by short periods of stage 2 NREM sleep.

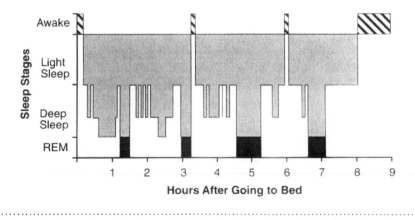

A typical night's sleep of a normal young adult. Notice how the sleep pattern shifts from stage to stage during the night.

The total amount of REM sleep during a normal night's sleep varies with age. Newborn babies spend about half of their sleeping time in REM sleep. By adulthood, REM sleep has decreased to about one-quarter of our total sleep time.

We all seem to need REM sleep, although nobody knows exactly why. The need may be related to REM dreaming, during which we seem to "process" the emotion-laden experiences of waking life.

In any case, our bodies appear to have an automatic mechanism that tries to obtain the normal amount of REM sleep for us. People who are deprived of REM sleep and then allowed to sleep normally usually experience several nights of what is called *REM rebound*, in which they spend an especially long time in REM sleep. It is as if their bodies sense that they have been deprived of REM sleep and are catching up on what was missed. People experiencing REM rebound tend to remember dreaming more and have more vivid and often scarier dreams than normal.

As you will see later in this chapter, people with sleep apnea are often deprived of the normal amount of REM sleep.

Normal Breathing During Sleep

Breathing Centers and Reflexes

Your breathing movements during sleep are controlled by automatic reflexes. These reflexes are driven by nervous system sensors, which constantly monitor the chemistry of your blood and send signals to the breathing centers of your brain. The breathing centers, in turn, send signals to your breathing muscles to regulate how fast and how powerfully you need to breathe at any particular time (see illustration at the top of page 34). This regulatory activity by the brain's breathing centers is one of the factors in the development of sleep apnea.

Sensors and "Set Points"

One group of sensors for monitoring your blood chemistry is in your carotid bodies, which are located in the carotid arteries in your neck. They sense the amount of oxygen in the blood that is on its way to your brain, and respond to low levels of oxygen in your blood. But even though oxygen is essential for life, particularly for your brain cells, these sensors are not the most important ones for your breathing reflex.

A more powerful set of sensors is in a deep and primitive part of your brain called the medulla. These sensors detect increases in the carbon dioxide in your cerebrospinal fluid (the fluid that bathes your brain and spinal cord). As your body uses up oxygen, it produces carbon dioxide, a waste gas. A high concentration of carbon dioxide in your cerebrospinal fluid signals that your body needs to breathe. When you breathe, you exhale carbon dioxide and immediately inhale fresh oxygen.

The particular concentration of carbon dioxide that triggers these sensors can be called the "set point." Whenever the carbon dioxide concentration rises high enough to

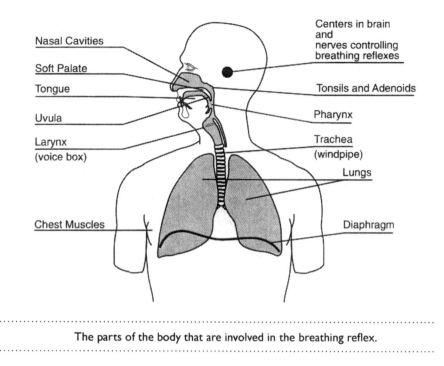

Nasal Cavities

Soft Palate

Tongue

Uvula

Larynx
(voice box)

Chest Muscles

Centers in brain
and
nerves controlling
breathing reflexes

Tonsils and Adenoids

Pharynx

Trachea
(windpipe)

Lungs

Diaphragm

The parts of the body that are involved in the breathing reflex.

reach the set point, the breathing reflex is activated. The oxygen sensors probably work in a similar way, but their set points are not nearly as sensitive during sleep.

The set points that trigger your breathing reflexes can move up and down, depending on a number of factors, including whether you are awake or asleep. During sleep the set points do not have to be as sensitive to low oxygen and high carbon dioxide as they do when you are awake, because your sleeping body needs less oxygen, your breathing is shallower, and the air in your lungs is exchanged less vigorously. So as you pass from waking to sleeping to waking, the set points cycle up and down (5).

Even during sleep, the set points seem to change. For example, during REM sleep the breathing responses become less sensitive. More carbon dioxide is tolerated, and the oxygen concentration can sometimes drop extremely low during REM sleep before the breathing reflexes finally are triggered (5).

The sensitivity of the set points is another factor in the development of sleep apnea.

Breathing Muscles

The act of breathing requires the use of several muscle groups in a number of places: the diaphragm, the rib cage (the intercostal and other muscles that attach to the ribs), the soft palate, the tongue, the upper and lower pharynx (the throat area behind the mouth), and the larynx (voice box). When breathing is normal, the actions of these assorted muscles are carefully coordinated. For example, when you inhale, your rib muscles contract, your tongue muscles automatically stabilize the position of your tongue, and your soft palate muscles become taut to hold your airway open.

The coordination among these various muscle groups during breathing is another factor in the development of sleep apnea.

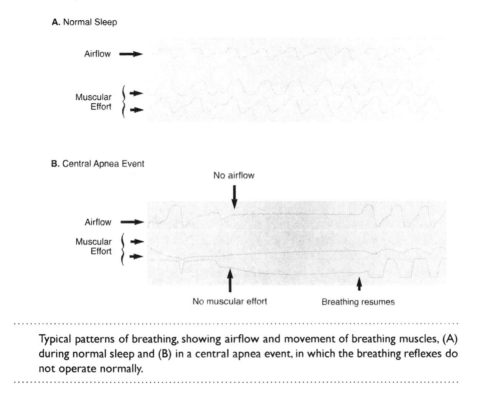

Typical patterns of breathing, showing airflow and movement of breathing muscles, (A) during normal sleep and (B) in a central apnea event, in which the breathing reflexes do not operate normally.

Snoring

Snoring occurs when your soft palate (the back part of the roof of your mouth) vibrates. A number of factors cause this. The muscle tone in your tongue and soft palate tends to decrease during sleep. They become more relaxed and can collapse together. This contributes to snoring. Other soft tissues, such as tonsils and tongue, can produce sounds that add to or change the quality of the snoring.

The position of the sleeper affects snoring. Lying on your back allows your tongue to fall back toward your throat and block your airway, so you are more likely to snore, and to snore the loudest, when you are lying on your back.

Anything that obstructs your airway will also contribute to snoring. For example, you are more likely to snore if you have large adenoids or a large tongue or if your nasal passages are swollen from a cold or allergies.

Weight gain can result in snoring because fatty tissue accumulates in the neck and can narrow the opening of the airway.

Age is also a factor. Older people tend to snore more because muscle tone tends to decrease with age.

Women are more likely to snore after menopause.

Other factors also aggravate snoring; alcoholic beverages, certain medications, and sheer physical exhaustion may be associated with heavy snoring.

Mere snoring, by itself, is not the same as sleep apnea. Many people snore without having the complete interruptions of breathing and sleep that are the signs of sleep apnea. Light or occasional snoring that does not interrupt breathing is not a health threat, although it can be a terrific annoyance to a sleeping partner. The solutions to harmless occasional snoring include the following:

Sleep on your side. You can train yourself to sleep on your side using a sleep position monitor (see Chapter 10).

Avoid alcohol before going to bed.

Check with your doctor to see whether any medication you are taking (either by prescription or over-the-counter) may be aggravating the snoring (see Chapter 10 and the Appendix).

If nasal congestion is a problem, ask your doctor about an antihistamine. You can consider using breathing nasal strips available in pharmacies.

Decrease your body weight.

The sleeping partner can wear soft foam earplugs when necessary. They are available from industrial safety stores and in many pharmacies.

When Simple Snoring Turns into Sleep Apnea

Snoring may turn into sleep apnea when the vibrations in the tongue and throat are accompanied by a number of other factors, discussed earlier in this chapter: an instability in the breathing reflexes, a structural narrowing of the airway (for example, from enlarged tonsils or weight gain), or a lack of coordination among the breathing muscles.

The severity of sleep-disordered breathing varies between individuals, and can become progressively worse. In some people, slight or occasional snoring may gradually develop into the heavy, more violent snoring that indicates sleep apnea. This process often begins in adolescence with heavy snoring and occasional short clusters of apnea events. Gradually, the picture may change to heavier snoring with longer sequences of nonbreathing. Later in adulthood, the pattern may evolve into obstructive apnea events that occur throughout nearly the whole night, with great disturbances in the structure of sleep, fluctuations in oxygen content of the blood, and daytime drowsiness (6). In some older people who have never had trouble with sleep apnea, the loss of muscle tone that occurs with age is enough to trigger the development of sleep apnea.

The reason snoring may progress to sleep apnea in some people and not in others depends on the sum of all the factors we have described here: breathing reflexes, structure of the airway, muscle coordination, and inherited tendencies.

◆ Summary

- The most important aspects of sleep are:
  - The quantity of sleep,
  - The quality of sleep
  - The amount of REM (rapid eye movement) sleep
- Sleep apnea interferes with all three of these.
- An abnormality in the breathing reflex during sleep can contribute to the development of sleep apnea.
- Snoring is caused by loss of muscle tone in the tongue and throat.
- Most of the sounds of typical snoring are caused by the vibration of the soft palate.
- Snoring in which breathing does not stop may be harmless. You may be able to decrease or eliminate this type of snoring by following suggestions in this chapter.

Snoring in which breathing stops is a symptom of sleep apnea.

7

What Causes Sleep Apnea?

- When someone has sleep apnea:
  - Breathing stops many times during sleep.
  - Oxygen in the blood stream decreases each time breathing stops.
  - The person wakes up many times to breathe during the night.
  - The result: not enough oxygen, and very poor sleep.
- Most people who have sleep apnea don't realize it.
- The sleeping partner usually is the first to notice sleep apnea.
- Heart disease and high blood pressure can be caused by the combination of the low oxygen levels, the strenuous efforts to breathe, and the sudden, repeated awakenings throughout the night.

A Typical Obstructive Sleep Apnea Event

CASE STUDY

Mr. Kennedy crawls into bed and turns out the light. He immediately falls asleep and begins to snore softly. His wife stuffs earplugs into her ears and wills herself to fall asleep quickly, before her husband really starts to snore. She reaches over and shakes his elbow.

"Roll over," she reminds him.

He complies, turns onto his side, and resumes his snoring.

Over the next few minutes, the sound of each snore becomes louder, more prolonged, more emphatic. Then all at once the room is silent. The snoring has stopped.

Is he still breathing? His ribs are moving in and out as though he is breathing, but no air is going in or out of his lungs. This is because the airway in his throat has collapsed shut while he is relaxed in sleep. His chest heaves in and out now, straining to breathe, even shaking the mattress with the force of the muscle contractions; but his throat is closed, so there still is no actual movement of air in and out.

Mr. Kennedy is suffocating.

This is obstructive apnea. Mr. Kennedy may struggle for a breath of air for as long as a minute, or even longer. Meanwhile, the oxygen supply in his body is running out and the carbon dioxide is accumulating.

Fortunately for Mr. Kennedy and the rest of our species, we all have a primitive, fail-safe, emergency arousal response. It awakens us at just such times as this and keeps us from suffocating during sleep. When Mr. Kennedy's arousal response finally is triggered, he wakes up. His body jerks and he gasps for air with a series of loud, snorting breaths, sucking oxygen into his lungs like a diver returning from the depths. This is the explosive snoring that is typical of sleep apnea.

In just a few seconds, fresh air pours into his lungs and the oxygen concentration in his blood reaches nearly normal, the carbon dioxide is expelled, and he returns to sleep. The arousal has been so brief that Mr. Kennedy is not aware of being awakened. He quickly returns to sleep, and the whole process will repeat itself.

Sleep Apnea Can Damage the Heart—And More

We need to pay attention to three important changes that took place in Mr. Kennedy's body during an apnea event:

1. When his emergency breathing reflex was triggered, his body experienced a surge in epinephrine (adrenalin), the *"fight-or-flight"* reflex, making his heart beat faster. These surges, repeated throughout the night, may eventually cause high blood pressure, even during daytime. High blood pressure increases the risk of stroke.
2. Each time Mr. Kennedy strained to breathe against the closed airway, sucking his rib cage inward, he made his heart work harder, pumping against that low pressure in order to send blood to his lungs and the rest of his body. This extreme pressure difference can cause enlargement of the heart, lung problems, and irregular heart rhythms. It may increase the chances that the heart will beat slower and slower and finally ... stop ... during sleep.
3. Finally, awakening to breathe again and again broke up the normal pattern of Mr. Kennedy's sleep. People with severe sleep apnea may never reach deep sleep; they have very fragmented REM sleep because of the constant arousals. Thus, throughout the night it is the deepest sleep that is most disturbed. Disturbed sleep leads to daytime drowsiness, sometimes so severe that it literally ruins a person's life. Automobile crashes are a common side effect of untreated sleep apnea.

The Three Types of Sleep Apnea

There are three kinds of sleep apnea, classified according to their causes: obstructive sleep apnea, central sleep apnea, and mixed apnea. The cause of the apnea determines treatment. Let's look at the cause of each type of sleep apnea.

Obstructive Sleep Apnea

In obstructive sleep apnea, the upper airway becomes blocked during sleep by the tissue of the soft palate, throat, and/or tongue. In Chapter 6, we explained that this blockage can result from a combination of anatomic factors and irregularities in the breathing reflex.

The person with obstructive sleep apnea struggles to breathe against an obstructed airway. His chest moves in and out but, because of the blockage, the air cannot flow into or out of his lungs. Finally, his oxygen concentration drops, as Mr. Kennedy's did, to the point where his arousal reflex causes him to breathe. He awakens with a loud, gasping, snorting sound.

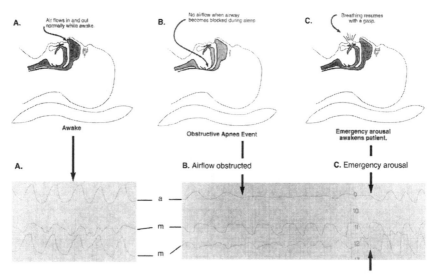

An obstructive apnea event. The polysomnographic recording shows airflow in and out of the airway (a) and the movements of the breathing muscles (m). A: Normal breathing while awake. B: The airway collapses and becomes obstructed during sleep. The breathing muscles continue to move, but no air can flow into the airway. C: Emergency arousal awakens the person, and he resumes breathing with a gasp.

People with obstructive apnea may have one or more anatomical abnormalities associated with their upper airway: the passages in their nose and pharynx (throat) (see illustration at the top of page 41). Such abnormalities can be seen in head radiograph images of many people with obstructive sleep apnea. (1).

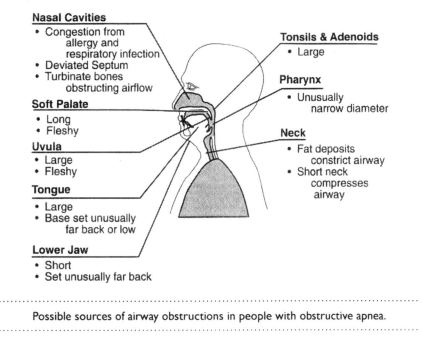

Nasal Cavities
- Congestion from allergy and respiratory infection
- Deviated Septum
- Turbinate bones obstructing airflow

Soft Palate
- Long
- Fleshy

Uvula
- Large
- Fleshy

Tongue
- Large
- Base set unusually far back or low

Lower Jaw
- Short
- Set unusually far back

Tonsils & Adenoids
- Large

Pharynx
- Unusually narrow diameter

Neck
- Fat deposits constrict airway
- Short neck compresses airway

Possible sources of airway obstructions in people with obstructive apnea.

In the nose, the abnormal structure may be a deviated nasal septum or chronic swelling of the nasal passages as a result of allergies.

In the upper pharynx, obstructions may include enlarged tonsils or adenoids, an extra-long or fleshy soft palate, or a large uvula (the fleshy tab that dangles in the back of your throat). In the lower pharynx, the problem might be a large tongue, a tongue that is located unusually far back or far down, an unusually small airway opening, a short lower jaw, or a short neck (1).

Any one of these structural features, or a combination of them, can help cause obstructive sleep apnea.

Body weight is often a factor in the development of obstructive apnea. One-half to three-fourths of patients with obstructive sleep apnea are more than 15 percent over their ideal weight (2). Obstructive sleep apnea is common in overweight people for several reasons. First, people who are carrying extra weight usually have fatty deposits within the throat tissue, which narrow the upper airway. Second, in some heavy people, the extra weight on the abdomen changes the way their stomach and chest muscles work, alters the operation of their breathing reflexes, and contributes to the development of apnea (see Chapter 11 for more on obesity and sleep apnea).

Age is also a factor in obstructive sleep apnea, because the shape and muscle tone of the upper airway tend to change with age. Many people have no sign of obstructive sleep apnea when they are younger but develop it in their 50s or 60s (see Chapter 15 for more about age and sleep apnea).

Gender is also a factor. Obstructive sleep apnea is approximately three times more prevalent among men. However, after menopause, a woman's tendency to develop obstructive sleep apnea increases dramatically.

Obstructive sleep apnea is treated by removing whatever is blocking the airway. This can be accomplished by means of a breathing device, or through surgery, and sometimes by both. If obesity is a factor, weight loss usually helps, if it can be maintained (see Chapter 10 for treatment of sleep apnea).

When a physician is seeking the cause of obstructive sleep apnea, it is extremely important to very carefully determine which of these many factors are contributing to the obstruction in order to choose the most effective treatment.

Central Sleep Apnea

Pure central apnea is the least common of the three types of sleep apnea. In central apnea, the cause of the breathing problem is in the brain, or central nervous system; thus, the term *central apnea*. In a person with central apnea, the respiratory center in the brain that controls breathing (described in Chapter 6) may simply stop working during sleep. It fails to signal the chest muscles to make breathing movements. Sleep researchers believe this may happen for a number of reasons, all related to some disorder in the breathing reflex. The disorder may be an inherited neurological problem or a neuromuscular disorder that arises later in life, such as, post-polio syndrome, muscular dystrophy, multiple sclerosis (MS), or amyotrophic lateral sclerosis (ALS, or Lou Gehrig's disease).

A person with pure central apnea has great difficulty sleeping and breathing at the same time. As soon as the person drops off to sleep, breathing stops (see illustration at the top of page 43). When the emergency arousal response takes over, the person awakens with a start and a gasp. In severe central apnea, the person may get very little sleep at all. This is an extremely distressing condition that can last for many years before it is correctly diagnosed.

Another form of central apnea is sometimes seen in people who have a psychological problem called sleep-onset anxiety. People with sleep-onset anxiety are panicky about falling asleep. This causes them to breathe quickly and heavily, which results in a decrease in the level of carbon dioxide in their blood. When they do fall asleep, the low carbon dioxide level fails to trigger their breathing reflex for a long time. Consequently, they end up having a central apnea event and awakening to breathe.

Typically, the main complaint of a person with central apnea is not getting enough sleep. He may describe his problem as "insomnia." The reason for his complaint, of course, is his frequent awakenings during the night. However, very few people with insomnia (only about 5 percent) have sleep apnea.

Obstruction of the airway usually is not a problem in a person with pure central apnea. However, research suggests that obstructive apnea sometimes can trigger central apnea (3). In these cases, the central apnea may disappear if the airway obstruction is treated.

People suffering from heart failure often have central sleep apnea. Their heart failure may improve once the central sleep apnea has been treated with continuous positive airway pressure (CPAP) (described in Chapter 10) (4).

The long-term effects of central apnea are similar to the effects of obstructive apnea: enlargement of the heart, lung complications, and heart failure.

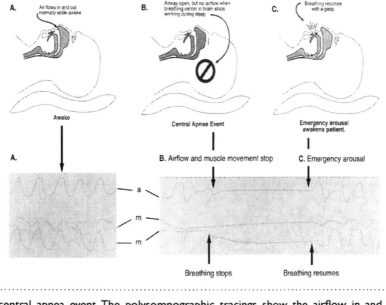

A central apnea event. The polysomnographic tracings show the airflow in and out of the airway (a) and the movement of the breathing muscles (m). A: Normal breathing while awake. B: Breathing movements and airflow stop during sleep. C: Emergency arousal awakens the person, and he resumes breathing with a gasp.

Bilevel positive airway pressure (bilevel PAP) is a treatment option for central sleep apnea. Drug therapy is a promising treatment. Other treatments might involve surgery, if there are airway obstructions, and possibly the use of a nighttime ventilating device. Pacemakers for the diaphragm have also been developed and may eventually be an acceptable treatment for central apnea. See Chapter 10 for more on treatment of sleep apnea.

Mixed Apnea

Mixed apnea is a combination of central and obstructive apnea. Most people with sleep apnea probably have some form of mixed apnea. In fact, some sleep researchers believe that most, if not all, obstructive sleep apnea has a central apnea component and that some abnormality in the breathing reflex in the brain usually accompanies the development of obstructive apnea.

Others interpret the cause and effect that occur in mixed apnea a little differently. They point out that as a person gasps and recovers from an obstructive apnea event, she typically "overbreathes," which results in an unusually low level of carbon dioxide in the blood. In turn, this lower carbon dioxide level is enough to trigger a central apnea event, thereby producing mixed apnea. The more severe the obstructive apnea, the more severe the "overbreathing" is likely to be and the more obvious the central apnea component could be.

In any case, whatever the actual cause and effect in mixed apnea, for treatment purposes, the obstructive apnea is usually treated first. Once the breathing obstruction is treated, the central apnea will often disappear, or at least lessen to the point where it does not require treatment.

◆ Summary

- Snoring in which breathing stops is a symptom of sleep apnea.
- Sleep apnea may cause cardiovascular problems and high blood pressure, and a higher risk of heart attack and stroke.
- There are three kinds of sleep apnea:
  - Central apnea, the least common type, originates in the brain.
  - Obstructive sleep apnea is caused by a blockage in the airway.
  - Mixed apnea, the most common type, is a combination of central and obstructive apnea.
- The choice of treatment depends on the kind of apnea.

Problems and Pitfalls of Identifying Sleep Apnea

- If you have a sleep problem, go to an accredited sleep disorders center. Locate the nearest to you at www.absm.org.
- Sleep apnea cannot be diagnosed by just talking with a doctor.
- You need an overnight sleep study to answer:
  - Do I have sleep apnea?
  - How severe is it?
  - How should it be treated?

Seeking the Correct Diagnosis

The first step in treating any medical problem is, of course, the correct diagnosis. To diagnose sleep apnea correctly, two important questions need to be answered:

1. Is this condition actually sleep apnea, or is it some other disorder?
2. Is sleep apnea the only disorder present, or are other conditions present that will complicate both the sleep apnea and the treatment?

The correct diagnosis of sleep apnea can be difficult for several reasons. Sleep apnea often is confused with a number of other sleep disorders, such as narcolepsy, insomnia, restless leg syndrome, or periodic limb movement in sleep. Or the opposite can occur: other disorders (heart conditions, breathing problems, seizure disorders) can be misdiagnosed as sleep apnea. Finally, sleep apnea can be hidden or aggravated by other factors, such as certain medications (sedatives, hypnotics, and beta blockers), alcohol, depression, heart disease, and obesity. For these reasons, it is important for someone with suspected sleep apnea to be thoroughly tested by a sleep specialist. Incorrect or mistaken treatment can be harmful.

Difficulties in Recognizing Sleep Apnea

The diagnosis of sleep disorders is a challenge. Unlike with most other diseases, a person may be completely unaware that he has a sleep disorder. Therefore, he may not be able to describe the most obvious symptoms because he is asleep when they occur. In some rare instances, a person will report a feeling that the throat is closing off during sleep, a feeling of choking on the tongue, or a feeling of gasping for breath during the night. Usually, however, people are completely unaware of any problem with breathing. Reports of breathing difficulties may come from a bed partner, roommate, or family member, but these descriptions can also underestimate the severity of the breathing problem.

Sleep specialists use a technology called polysomnography to confirm the diagnosis of sleep apnea and other sleep disorders. Other methods of diagnosing sleep disorders, such as questionnaires, have been tried in the past, but are not accurate enough to recognize particular sleep disorders or estimate severity.

Polysomnography is the electronic measurement of sleep. It consists of using electronic monitors to record the patient's physiological signals during a full night's sleep, and then analyzing the recording of the electronic signals. Until these tools became available, sleep apnea went unrecognized.

Appropriately used, polysomnographic testing can distinguish between sleep disorders and other conditions and can measure their severity. Polysomnography is described in detail in Chapter 9.

Even with these modern tools, however, sleep apnea can be misdiagnosed. Inappropriate sleep testing can lead to incorrect diagnosis and treatment. Tests must be done according to established standards; otherwise, the test results may be faulty. For example, testing for sleep apnea by means of daytime naps or a partial night's sleep may give a false picture. Daytime sleep is qualitatively different from nighttime sleep. Because sleep apnea often is worse during the second half of the night, when most REM sleep occurs, a partial night sleep test may underestimate the severity of sleep apnea. Also, if the person sleeps poorly during a test, he may appear to have little or no apnea. Sleep apnea may actually improve with disturbed sleep and appear less severe because the person is in a lighter stage of sleep, so that the healthy, "awake" breathing center is more active than it is during a usual night's sleep.

Another reason sleep apnea has been difficult to diagnose is that most medical people are not very familiar with the condition. Only in the 1980s did doctors begin to recognize sleep apnea as a specific sleep/breathing disorder with characteristic causes and symptoms. It is still best understood by sleep specialists. Even today, the average medical student receives only about 24 minutes of instruction on sleep disorders during his or her entire medical education (1).

Unless your doctor is a recent graduate of one of the few medical schools that teach about sleep disorders, his or her only contact with the field may be the medical literature, which contains an occasional article about sleep disorders. Reading about sleep apnea is not the same as recognizing the symptoms in a patient. The diagnostic routines that most doctors learn in medical school never prompt them to look for the symptoms of sleep apnea.

A typical sequence of treatment begins when a physician fails to recognize the sleep apnea and attempts to treat the symptoms. Complaints of snoring, excessive day-time sleepiness (EDS), unexplained fatigue, and/or "insomnia" should be clear signals of possible sleep apnea. Instead these symptoms often are treated with drugs, such as stimulants or sleeping medications, and the underlying sleep apnea is missed or even aggravated, sometimes for many years.

Another common sequence of treatment begins when a patient first talks with a surgeon to try to solve his snoring problem. The surgeon fails to refer the patient for proper sleep testing and does a little snoring surgery on a hunch that "you don't have sleep apnea." The snoring may improve for a while, but if the person has underlying sleep apnea, it remains undetected and untreated. The American Academy of Otolaryngology (ear, nose, and throat surgeons) has published guidelines that require patients with snor-ing to be properly tested before they have snoring surgery. Yet, some surgeons still believe they can tell if someone has significant apnea by simply talking to the person!

If sleep apnea is not diagnosed or treated properly, it may become severe enough that heart and lung complications appear, as in the case of Reverend. Allen (described in Chapter 1). Even then, many physicians will continue to treat the symptoms without suspecting that a sleep/breathing disorder may be the cause.

The difficulties in diagnosing sleep apnea have led to an enormous amount of frustration. Sick people go from doctor to doctor, for years, continuing to suffer from the symptoms of sleep apnea, desperately seeking an answer. People have died, and many more have reached the brink of death, before a chance encounter (a spouse, a friend, a news article, a change of physicians) finally has brought them to a sleep center for proper testing and a clear diagnosis of sleep apnea.

Avoiding Misdiagnosis

The following are 10 rules for avoiding misdiagnosis:

1. *Select an accredited sleep center and be evaluated by a physician who has specialized in sleep disorders.*

How can you know if the sleep center and the physician are accredited? Call the American Academy of Sleep Medicine (AASM) and ask them for the nearest accredited sleep specialist or sleep center, or find a list of accredited sleep centers on their web site at www.aasmnet.org. Or you can ask whether a particular sleep laboratory has been accredited by the AASM or whether a particular physician is "board certified" as a specialist in sleep disorders (see also Chapter 16).

If you live in an area without an accredited sleep laboratory, or if you belong to an HMO that is not associated with an accredited sleep center, you may be able to find a good sleep laboratory that is not accredited. In that case, ask your HMO or your state medical society to refer you to a physician who has had formal training in the treatment of sleep apnea. Ask for evidence that you are being treated by a physician who is trained in sleep disorders. If it is clear that your HMO does not have access to a trained physician, consider appealing to the administration and obtain a referral to the nearest accredited sleep laboratory.

Accreditation is the consumer's best signpost for locating a competent sleep center. A physician earns accreditation in sleep disorders medicine by passing a rigorous examination. To be sure you are being treated by someone who is a certified sleep expert, ask the following question: "Have you passed the examination for sleep specialists given by the American Board of Sleep Medicine?" If you are hesitant about asking your doctor this question directly, you can telephone his office and ask his receptionist the question. If she does not know the answer, ask her to find out and call you back.

CASE STUDY

Mr. Woods was seen at his HMO and told that he needed a sleep study. He was assured that the HMO had a "sleep lab" and that a "sleep expert" would diagnose his problem. After a night in the sleep lab, he was told that he had central sleep apnea and was discouraged to learn that not much could be done for him.

Later, Mr. Woods was studied in an accredited sleep center, where he was found to have idiopathic central nervous system (CNS) hypersomnolence, not central apnea. He also had mild sleep apnea, but it was obstructive rather than central. With medications for his idiopathic CNS hypersomnolence, he was able to return to work, and with weight loss, the obstructive apnea disappeared.

CASE STUDY

Mr. Costello heard about sleep apnea and realized that he had several symptoms: heavy snoring, a weight problem, and falling asleep while driving. He discussed this with his family doctor, who gave him a continuous positive airway pressure (CPAP) machine and told him to go home and use it on a setting of "6."

Mr. Costello tried sleeping with the CPAP, but kept waking up feeling suffocated and struggling with the mask. After a week of fiddling with the CPAP setting and the mask, he gave up in frustration and returned the CPAP to the doctor's office.

A few months later, Mr. Costello fell asleep at the wheel, crashed his car, and injured himself. He was referred to an accredited sleep center for a sleep study and was diagnosed with severe sleep apnea. This time the sleep center fitted him properly with a CPAP mask and custom-set the prescribed CPAP pressure for him in the sleep laboratory. He was surprised to find that he could sleep well with the CPAP, and within a few weeks he felt better than he had in years.

2. *Be sure that your sleep study is performed at night or during your usual sleep hours.*

If you are told to "stay awake all night and then come into the laboratory in the morning to have your sleep test," find another sleep center.

If you are a shift worker and are accustomed to sleeping during the day, either have your study during the day or switch back to sleeping at night for at least three nights before going into the laboratory for a sleep study at night.

CASE STUDY

Mr. Daly was told to stay up all night and then come into the sleep lab to have a sleep study. He slept poorly in the lab, and after three hours he had to end the study because he couldn't sleep any longer. He was diagnosed as having some sleep apnea and told to lose weight.

Later, he was restudied properly in a nighttime sleep test at an accredited sleep center. He was found to have severe sleep apnea, particularly during the last 4 hours of the night, which the earlier sleep study had missed because it did not examine Mr. Daly during his usual sleep hours.

Appropriate treatment included not only weight loss but also uvulopalatophar yngoplasty (UPPP) surgery and the use of CPAP (see Chapter 10). With treatment, Mr. Daly improved remarkably and eventually was even able to discontinue CPAP.

3. *If you are sleepy while driving and working, be sure that a Multiple Sleep Latency Test (MSLT) is performed on the day following your nighttime sleep study.*

An MSLT will establish the severity of your daytime sleepiness. It also will help rule out other causes of sleepiness (for example, other sleep disorders) and provide a baseline to refer to if fatigue and sleepiness continue after the apnea has been treated.

CASE STUDY

Ms. Jones snored frequently and heavily, and had felt tired for years. She was sleepy when driving and couldn't stay awake during her favorite operas. She went to a "sleep lab" and was told she needed UPPP surgery.

After surgery, she was pleased that she no longer snored, felt better, and was not sleepy while driving. However, she still felt tired. She was told that her trouble was related to stress and boredom.

She was restudied at an accredited sleep center, and her sleep study showed that despite the surgery, she still had most of her sleep apnea. It also uncovered a second major sleep disorder that previously had been missed —narcolepsy.

4. *Be sure that you have had a recent thorough physical examination and laboratory studies, preferably with your own physician, who knows your past health problems and has all your records available.*

This will avoid duplication of tests.

Mr. Roberts was told that sleep apnea was the cause of his snoring and progressive fatigue. He had gained weight, so he was put on a weight-loss program and referred to a surgeon for UPPP surgery.

He obtained a second opinion at an accredited sleep center, and physical examination found that he had low thyroid activity. Treatment eliminated his fatigue. He quickly lost the extra weight, which had also been caused by his thyroid disorder, and his apnea then disappeared.

5. *Be sure you have a thorough examination of your throat, preferably by an ear, nose, and throat specialist (also known as an ENT specialist, or otolaryngologist) who is experienced with sleep apnea.*

Mr. Wilson had been told by his doctor that he probably had sleep apnea, but the doctor wouldn't refer him to a sleep center unless he lost weight. Six months later, Mr. Wilson felt worse and obtained a referral from another physician.

He was found to have mild apnea, and an ENT specialist examined his throat and found a cancer narrowing his lower throat area. Mr. Wilson then realized he had been having a little trouble swallowing food, but he had not considered it to be enough of a problem to mention.

6. *If CPAP is recommended, be sure you are studied with CPAP in the sleep laboratory, so that the proper air pressure can be established to control your obstructive apnea.*

This may mean spending a second night in the sleep testing laboratory. If CPAP is prescribed for you and you are simply told to "go home and try it out," find another sleep center.

Ms. Brown had heart problems, and her blood oxygen levels were checked during an evaluation for chest pain, but sleep studies were not done. Because she snored, she was told that sleep apnea was the cause of the decrease in oxygen in her blood while sleeping. She was told to go home and use CPAP.

She slept very poorly with CPAP, but she was told to keep using it because her blood oxygen was much better.

Too frightened to stop using CPAP but exhausted from not sleeping, she was studied at an accredited sleep center. She was found to have very mild apnea, but it was central apnea, not obstructive apnea, and could not be treated effectively with CPAP.

7. *If surgery, oral devices, medications, or weight loss are prescribed for you, be sure to have a sleep study to establish a baseline, so that it can be determined whether you are benefiting from the treatment, and if so how much.*

People often feel better after treatment begins, and think they are "cured" when, in fact, they may be only partially improved. Further treatment or careful follow-up may be necessary.

CASE STUDY

Mr. Johnson was diagnosed with severe obstructive sleep apnea. He had UPPP surgery and stopped snoring. His wife said he was cured because she "didn't notice any more apnea." Mr. Johnson felt "much better." He was told by the surgeon that a follow-up sleep study was not necessary since he obviously was cured.

Mr. Johnson's family doctor noticed that his blood pressure had not improved and convinced him to return to the sleep center. His follow-up sleep study showed that he had only improved 25 percent. The following night he was placed on CPAP. He improved more than he could have believed, and his blood pressure dropped so far that his family doctor was able to stop one of his medications.

8. *If you are diagnosed as having obstructive apnea but you believe that you have other reasons for feeling tired or drowsy or for having restless sleep, be sure to discuss them with your physician. It is possible that sleep apnea may not be the most important cause of your symptoms.*

A trial with CPAP in the sleep laboratory is a good way to find out how many of your problems are caused by sleep apnea. CPAP safely eliminates any sleep apnea that you may have, and you can then be the judge of whether you feel better or still have troublesome symptoms. If you are in doubt about how important sleep apnea is in causing your drowsiness, return to the laboratory for a trial with CPAP.

The opposite is also true: you may believe that you have fairly serious sleep apnea symptoms even though your sleep test may say that your apnea is too mild for treatment. If this is the case, you may be one of those individuals who is very sensitive to sleep disruption from apnea. Discuss this possibility with your doctor. A trial with CPAP would be very helpful in letting you judge how much improvement you feel after the apnea is eliminated.

9. *If sleep studies show that your apnea is well controlled but you continue to be sleepy, feel fatigued, or experience sleep disturbances, be sure that your doctor has considered and ruled out other conditions that might be causing those symptoms.*

As many as 20 percent of patients with sleep apnea have other undiagnosed sleep disorders that may not be obvious until the sleep apnea is diagnosed.

10. *Be sure that stress factors, depression, sleep habits, and drug and alcohol use have been thoroughly discussed with you.*

Unless the physician carefully questions you about these areas, they may continue to be problems that neither you nor your doctor fully understands! Two case studies show how unexpected factors can strongly affect the results of treatment for sleep apnea.

CASE STUDY

Mr. Williams was sent by his heart specialist to have a "sleep study." He was not seen by a sleep specialist but was told that he had significant sleep apnea, which caused his broken sleep, chronic fatigue, headaches, and drowsiness. He was sent to have UPPP surgery, and the surgeon recommended that he go to an accredited sleep center for reevaluation.

The sleep specialist discovered that Mr. Williams was very depressed and had been hiding the extent of his drug and alcohol use. Mr. Williams agreed to have drug and alcohol treatment and eventually was treated with antidepressants and counseling. His sleep disorder resolved, and a sleep study showed that he had such mild apnea that further treatment was not necessary. His alcohol use and depression had aggravated his apnea and sleep-related symptoms.

CASE STUDY

Mr. Jones went through a divorce and became depressed. He gained a lot of weight and eventually was diagnosed as having severe sleep apnea. CPAP helped somewhat, but to the dismay of both Mr. Jones and his doctor, he had no luck losing his excess weight.

Mr. Jones was still having problems with depression and finally went to see a psychiatrist. As counseling progressed and his depression lifted, he began to lose weight. He eventually had UPPP surgery, his remaining mild apnea and snoring disappeared, and he was even able to discontinue CPAP.

In Mr. Jones's case, neither his sleep apnea nor his weight gain was likely to improve very much until he was treated for depression.

What Should You Do If You Think You Have Sleep Apnea?

If you think you have sleep apnea:

1. *First try working through your family doctor. Make an appointment and tell him or her that you think you have sleep apnea and why you think so. Ask for a referral to an accredited sleep center to be tested for sleep apnea.*

When you see your family doctor, take with you any articles or books that have helped convince you that you have sleep apnea. You might also take along a tape recording of your snoring.

If your doctor doesn't "hear" you (that is, he is not familiar with sleep apnea or does not take your diagnosis seriously) and you are still convinced you are right, proceed to step 2.

2. *Call the nearest accredited sleep center yourself (see the preceding section and Chapter 16. Ask for an appointment. Some sleep centers will take patients only by referral from another physician, but many centers will make appointments with patients directly. If you are in an HMO, ask your primary care physician for a referral to an accredited sleep specialist. If denied, appeal and appeal again. You might use this book to back up your appeal.*

It is always best to work with your family doctor. If you decide to contact a sleep center directly, it still is a good idea to keep your family doctor informed. For one thing, he probably will become involved eventually because the sleep clinic will probably contact him to get your medical history. Later, as a courtesy, they probably will notify him or her of the treatment they recommend for you. In fact, depending on the kind of treatment, your family doctor may need to become actively involved. In addition, keeping your family doctor informed will expose him or her to more experience with sleep apnea, which will help other people with sleep apnea in the future.

Keep in mind that it is your health that is at stake. If your doctor seems uncooperative, you should not hesitate to get in touch with a sleep center yourself.

If the closest accredited sleep center only accepts referrals and your doctor is unwilling to refer you, take the next step.

3. *Ask the sleep center for one of the following:*
   a. The name of a local doctor with whom they have worked who will refer you to the sleep clinic
   b. The location of the closest qualified sleep center that will accept patients without a doctor's referral

The next chapter takes you to a sleep clinic.

◆ Summary

- Sleep apnea is frequently mistaken for other conditions.
- Misdiagnosis results in incorrect treatment, sometimes with disastrous consequences.
- A specialist in sleep disorders medicine at an accredited sleep center is the physician most likely to correctly test for and diagnose sleep apnea.
- The American Academy of Sleep Medicine (AASM) can put you in touch with the nearest accredited sleep specialist or sleep center.

■ The 10 rules for avoiding misdiagnosis and the "What Should You Do . . . ?" sections of this chapter will guide you toward an accurate diagnosis.

9

The Sleep Center: Testing for Sleep Apnea

The Full-Service Sleep Center

Polysomnography

Sleep specialists have developed a standard way to record and measure what is going on during a person's sleep. The procedure is called polysomnography, which means "making multiple sleep recordings." The electronic apparatus that is used is called (not too surprisingly) a polysomnograph.

If you have ever had an electrocardiogram (ECG or EKG) or an electroencephalogram (EEG), or if you have ever seen the way a lie detector test (polygraph) is performed, you know exactly the kind of equipment that is used for polysomnography.

A polysomnograph records a person's sleep by gathering information from a set of small electrodes glued to the patient's skin. Wires lead from the electrodes to a computer, which translates the electrical signals into squiggly lines on a computer screen (see illustration at the top of page 55). The procedure runs all night and records all the information from a full night's sleep.

To study a person's sleep, each of the electrodes is attached with tape or a dab of glue to a specific location on the person's skin. The electrodes usually are placed on the following places:

Head, as for an EEG, to record brain wave activity that distinguishes the stages of sleep and wakefulness
Face near the outside corner of each eye to detect eye movements
Chin or throat to detect jaw muscle tone
Chest to pick up signals of the heartbeat, as in an ECG
Abdomen to detect abdominal movements
Legs to detect abnormal leg movements

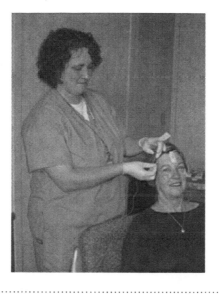

A patient being prepared for a sleep test.

Each of these electrodes picks up information about a particular activity going on during sleep. The recordings from each electrode can then be analyzed by comparing them with standardized "normal" recordings.

When sleep apnea is being studied, several additional recordings are made to gather information about the person's breathing and to show when air is moving in and out of the airway.

One recording wire is attached to a stretchy belt that contains a device that is fastened around the person's chest to detect expansion and contraction of the rib cage and abdomen as the muscles make breathing movements.

Another recording device is a pulse oximeter, which is clipped gently onto a finger or earlobe. The oximeter measures the oxygen content in the person's blood. It works by shining light through the skin into the capillaries, where the hemoglobin in the blood absorbs the light. Hemoglobin carries oxygen, so the amount of light absorbed shows how much oxygen is in the blood.

- Another device measures air moving in and out through the nose and mouth. This is done using a small detector that rests lightly on the upper lip just beneath the nose.

In some cases, additional monitors may be used to detect other types of sleep-disordered breathing.

Once all the electrodes and other recording devices are attached to the person being studied, the wires are gathered together into a "pigtail" to keep them out of the way and avoid restricting freedom of movement. The bundle of wires plugs into a box, which leads to an adjacent room, where the bulk of the polysomnographic equipment is located.

It is important to emphasize that nothing about this recording procedure hurts! There are no needles or other pain-causing devices. The electrodes are simply stuck to the skin with adhesive. Since they are only measuring a person's own biological activity, they will not cause an electrical shock.

The sleep study takes place in a private sleep room, which is supplied with a comfortable bed. The sleep room is very well insulated so that all outside sounds and lights are screened out, and nothing can disturb the person's sleep. The room is kept at a temperature that is comfortable for sleeping. Some sleep centers make the sleep rooms "homey," with carpeting, drapes, and pictures on the walls, whereas other sleep rooms look more like hospital rooms.

The Job of the Sleep Technician

Sleep technicians hook you up to the polysomnography leads, make you comfortable during the night, and monitor both your sleep and the operation of the polysomnograph equipment throughout the night. The accuracy of the results of your sleep study will depend on how well the technicians do their job, so their skill and diligence are very important.

Sleep technicians may have a wide range of training and experience, from beginners who are receiving "hands-on" training to well-trained experts who have taken courses in their field and keep up-to-date on the latest information on sleep testing and measurement techniques.

A sign of proficiency in this field is the credential of Registered Polysomnographic Technologist (RPSGT). Sleep technicians can earn this credential by training, studying, and passing a comprehensive 2-day test administered by the Board of Registered Polysomnographic Technologists.

In most well-staffed sleep centers, at least the supervisor of the sleep technicians will be an RPSGT. It is important that the person in charge of the actual sleep testing have thorough understanding of the standardized procedures for setting up and carrying out a valid sleep test. Supervision by an RPSGT gives some assurance that polysomnographic equipment will be connected to the patient according to the accepted standards and that the sleep recordings will be accurate. Poorly conducted sleep tests can produce recordings that look accurate and impressive but lead to an incorrect diagnosis and may need to be repeated later on. Thus, bad sleep tests not only are a waste of your time and money, but also can actually result in bad medical treatment.

A Visit to a Sleep Center

Let's assume that you suspect you may have sleep apnea. Your first contact with a sleep center will probably be something like Mr. Kennedy's.

Mrs. Kennedy said, "Honey, please do something about that snoring," so he made an initial appointment with the sleep specialist at the nearest accredited sleep center. His wife was asked to come along with her husband to the initial discussion with the doctor.

This is the usual procedure. It's helpful for both partners to be present because the sleeping partner probably will be able to supply more information about the person's sleep than the sleeper himself or herself. In addition, sleep disturbances such as sleep apnea frequently require long-term treatment, which affects both partners in some ways, so it is a good idea for both to be part of the process from the very beginning.

At the end of Mr. Kennedy's initial interview, the sleep specialist told him that he suspected sleep apnea and advised him to make an appointment for evaluation during an all-night sleep session.

He was scheduled for a date 2 weeks later to spend a night at the sleep center. He was told to plan also to spend part of the following day there for further testing. Sometimes patients spend two nights in the sleep center, but not the day in between. The testing schedule depends on the policies and procedures of the particular sleep center.

On the day of Mr. Kennedy's all-night sleep session, he was asked to arrive at the sleep center in the evening, a little before his normal bedtime, so the technician would have plenty of time to attach the electrodes and other recording devices to him. Most sleep centers ask people to avoid alcohol, narcotics, and caffeine during the day before their sleep test to eliminate any chance that these substances will interfere with sleep.

Although he knew there was nothing painful about the procedure of recording sleep, Mr. Kennedy admits to feeling some anxiety as he arrived at the sleep center. He is not alone in feeling anxious; many people are uneasy when facing an unfamiliar medical procedure.

Mr. Kennedy was told that he could wear his own nightclothes as long as they fit loosely and did not interfere with the placement of the electrodes. He brought a pair of pajamas, which worked fine.

When the measuring devices had all been attached, Mr. Kennedy was able to read a book or watch TV until his normal bedtime. Then the technician came in and turned out the lights and left him to go to sleep. The technician gave him a buzzer to use in case he needed to get up during the night to use the bathroom or needed to have the technician help him with something. Then the technician would come in and unplug his polysomnograph wires.

At any time while you are at the sleep center, be sure to tell the nurses or technicians if you feel nervous whenever you are undergoing any kind of medical procedure.

The medical personnel want you to be at ease. Feel free to ask questions if you are alarmed or even just curious. The technicians who prepare you for your night of sleep are so familiar with the routine that they may forget to explain the details as clearly as they should. It is okay to remind them that you are new at this and would like to understand what is going on. Everything should be clearly explained to you.

CASE STUDY

M r. Kennedy did buzz the technician once during the night. When it seemed as though a long time had passed and the technician had not appeared, Mr. Kennedy simply unclipped the oxygen sensor from his finger. The sudden change in the signal on the polysomnographic recording told the technician that Mr. Kennedy's blood oxygen signal had disappeared. The technician arrived instantly to reattach the sensor.

Mr. Kennedy worried that he would never get to sleep with so many wires attached to his body. But the next thing he knew, the technician was waking him up and telling him it was morning.

Despite the unfamiliar setting, most people manage to get a fairly decent night's sleep.

You may be asked to stay for part of the next day to take a multiple sleep latency test (MSLT). Sleep latency is a measure of how long it takes a person to fall asleep during the daytime. It indicates the degree of excessive daytime sleepiness (EDS) the person is experiencing. As you already know, EDS is one of the symptoms of sleep apnea.

To measure sleep latency, you will simply be asked to return to the sleep room several times during the day for 20-minute rest periods, while the polysomnograph records whether you fall asleep and exactly how long it takes to do so.

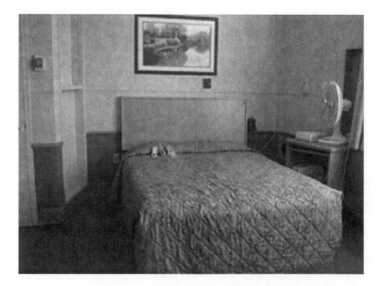

A comfy sleep room in a sleep center.

You will be detached from the recorder between MSLT naps and will be free to walk around, read, watch television, or even go to the cafeteria for lunch. Of course, you will still have all your electrodes attached and a clump of wires dangling around your neck. Some people are not bothered a bit by this. Others, like Mr. Kennedy, feel a little like Frankenstein's monster and prefer to have lunch delivered so they do not have to wander very far from the sleep center.

If you are staying in the sleep center for an MSLT, be sure to bring along something to entertain yourself: a book or magazine, crossword puzzles, needlework, or a deck of cards. If you object to wandering around in your bathrobe all day, you might bring some loose-fitting day-wear, such as a caftan or a jogging suit, which can be comfortably worn over the wires.

After all the recordings are completed, the doctor will read through the record of your sleep night, looking for signs that indicate whether you have sleep apnea, and, if so, what kind and how severe it is. Another appointment will be scheduled for you to discuss the results and, if necessary, the treatment options.

The "Split-Night" Sleep Study

The standard way to diagnose and treat sleep apnea requires two full nights in the sleep laboratory. The first night is for a diagnostic sleep study. If the sleep specialist diagnoses sleep apnea and prescribes the most common treatment, CPAP (continuous positive airway pressure) (see Chapter 10), the patient spends a second full night in the sleep laboratory so that the CPAP pressure can be custom set for him or her.

In some cases, this two-night procedure is compressed into one night. This is called a "split-night" sleep study. If the patient shows signs of sleep apnea during the first half of the night, CPAP treatment is begun and the CPAP pressure is custom set during the second half of the night.

Split-night studies have two major advantages: first, one night in the sleep laboratory is less expensive than two nights; and second, the sleep laboratory can test more patients by doing split-night studies.

However, a split-night study has several important disadvantages: it can fail to accurately show the severity of the apneas. Sleep apnea usually is worse during REM sleep, which occurs mostly during the second half of the night. If a doctor is basing a diagnosis on apneas observed only during the first half of the night, he may underestimate the seriousness of a patient's sleep apnea. This is especially likely in patients who have split-night studies and are told that they have "moderate" apnea. The split-night study may miss the true severity of their apnea when sleeping in certain positions or during REM. Later, if CPAP fails to treat the patient, the insurer may refuse additional treatment, claiming that the apnea is only mild. Other problems occur when a split-night study results in diagnosing a severe sleep apnea patient as being mild or moderate, and after CPAP fails they want to consider surgery. The surgeon may be misled by the findings of mild apnea and make ill-advised surgical recommendations. If you have a split-night study, carefully consider a full diagnostic study before having surgery.

Another possible disadvantage of a split-night study is that, even though the patient may have sleep apnea that needs treatment, the split-night may not produce enough information to convince an insurance company to pay for treatment.

Finally, there may not be enough time during the second half of the night to obtain an accurate CPAP pressure. For this reason, the American Academy of Sleep Medicine does not consider split-night studies appropriate for all patients.

At-Home Sleep Testing: Portable Monitoring

Under certain conditions, it is not necessary to spend a night in a sleep disorders center. In-home testing for sleep disorders (also called portable monitoring or ambulatory monitoring) is a new and developing field. For certain patients, and under certain conditions, the sleep specialist may suggest that the sleep study be done in the person's home.

Having a sleep study in your own home might sound to you like a better idea than spending the night in a strange place that reminds you of a hospital. Some proponents of in-home testing claim that people's sleep is more "normal" during an in-home test than in the sleep laboratory. However, there is no clear evidence to prove this, or to prove that in-home testing is necessarily more comfortable for the patient. For some people, an in-home test may have numerous drawbacks. Sleep may be disturbed by other family members, by the home surroundings, by neighborhood noises, and by other interruptions that are not present in a sleep center. On the other hand, a sleep center has a carefully regulated environment and trained technicians available in case problems arise. Furthermore, sleep specialists take into account the strangeness of the setting—called the "first night effect"—when they analyze the data from your sleep study in the sleep laboratory.

There are other important differences between an in-laboratory study and an in-home study. Your sleep specialist will consider these differences when deciding where you should have your sleep study.

Let's compare the two kinds of sleep studies (see Table at top of page 61).

When considering an in-home sleep study, you need to ask two questions:

1. What kind of in-home testing will be used?
2. For which patients is in-home testing appropriate, and are you one of them?

What Kind of In-Home Testing Is Used for Sleep Apnea Diagnosis?

In-home sleep studies vary widely in many ways. The apparatus itself can range from very simple to very complicated: from a single sensor that records the amount of oxygen in the blood to a complete "12-lead" arrangement much like polysomnography that is done in a sleep laboratory. How the in-home study is set up varies from one sleep laboratory to another. Sometimes the patient goes to the doctor's office and takes the apparatus home with him or her. Sometimes a technician comes to the patient's home and sets up the equipment.

In 1994, the American Sleep Disorders Association (today called the American Academy of Sleep Medicine, AASM) published its first set of recommendations on

Comparison of In-Lab and In-Home Sleep Studies		
	In-Lab Study, Accredited Sleep Center	In-Home
Technology	Well developed	Newer
Standards exist?	Yes	Yes
Technician training	Good	Varies from good to none
Cost	Higher	Lower
Accuracy	Good	Good to poor
Chance for errors	Low	High
Need to repeat study because of errors	Rare	Common
Paid for by insurance?	Yes	Often no

the standards and practices for portable sleep testing (1). For diagnosing sleep apnea, the association's committee of sleep specialists recommended that at least four types of measurements (four "leads") are needed. Two leads should record breathing (breathing movements and/or airflow), and there should be one lead each for heart rate (or ECG) and oxygen in the blood. It is not good enough to measure just blood oxygen, as the simplest studies do.

Notice that with only four leads, *no information is recorded about actual sleep or sleep stages* because brain waves are not monitored. In a patient with less severe apnea, data on sleep and sleep stages often are considered necessary for diagnosing sleep apnea. This is why a person with less serious sleep apnea symptoms may need to go to a sleep laboratory for a complete, polysomnographic sleep study, while, paradoxically, a patient with more severe symptoms may be diagnosed by a simpler sleep study at home.

Whether the sleep study is "attended" or "unattended" is another issue. Some in-home studies are attended, which means either that a technician remains in the home to monitor the study or that the patient is monitored remotely by the sleep laboratory, so that if something goes wrong, the sleep laboratory technician knows immediately and can call the patient's home and solve the problem. Many things can go wrong during a sleep study. Equipment has been known to fail during the night, and it is not unusual for movements during sleep to cause electrodes to come loose from the patient's skin. If no technician is present to fix the problem, the results of the sleep study may be worthless. Studies that are unattended may need to be repeated if something goes wrong during the night. Repeating sleep studies is expensive, which explains why some insurance providers are reluctant to pay for in-home sleep studies. The AASM guidelines recommend that all sleep studies be attended studies (2).

Another issue with in-home sleep testing is the training and skill of the staff carrying out the test. A test set up by a poorly trained technician or analyzed by an unqualified person may generate misleading results. The AASM standards specify that only a licensed physician may order an in-home sleep test, and that the individuals who set up and evaluate the test should be certified or eligible for certification. However, at present, the consumer has no assurances about the training or qualifications of technicians conducting in-home studies.

For Which Patients Is In-Home Testing Appropriate?

The 1994 recommendations by the AASM suggest that in-home testing may be appropriate in the following cases:

1. For patients who have obvious, severe symptoms and seem very likely to have sleep apnea (habitual snoring, excessive daytime sleepiness, obesity, and observed apneas), an in-home study can be used basically to confirm the diagnosis of sleep apnea in order to start treatment as soon as possible.
2. An in-home or portable study may be used for patients who cannot get to a sleep laboratory because they either are too ill to be moved or live too far away from a sleep disorders center.
3. For a follow-up sleep study, after a patient has been diagnosed and treated for a while, an in-home test sometimes can be used to see whether the treatment has been effective.

If an in-home sleep study is suggested to you, ask how many measurements will be recorded. Will there be at least four leads, as recommended by the AASM? Do not accept assurances lightly.

Unless you have very obvious sleep apnea (habitual snoring, excessive daytime sleepiness, obesity, and observed apneas) that just needs to be confirmed, you should make sure that the sleep study will actually monitor your **sleep**, not just your heart rate or your blood oxygen level. This means that sensors should be attached to your head to monitor brain waves (electroencephogram, EEG), eye movements (electro-oculogram, EOG), and chin movements (electromyography, EMG) as well as heart rate, breathing or airflow, oxygen saturation, and body movements.

In-home testing has some strong advocates. Among these are some small sleep laboratories that are not equipped to test large numbers of patients. The ability to test patients at home is an advantage for such laboratories.

Homecare providers and medical equipment manufacturers are also expanding into the business of in-home testing. Generally, they supply the equipment, send a technician to the patient's home to set up the test, and send the results to a physician for analysis. The AASM recommends against any arrangement in which the company conducting the test stands to profit from the results by selling the patient a CPAP unit or homecare services. The possibility for conflict of interest here is obvious.

Unless and until professional standards such as those recommended by the AASM are agreed upon and followed, in-home testing can be expected to vary widely in its accuracy and cost-effectiveness.

Determining the Severity of Sleep Apnea

When is a person's sleep apnea severe enough to cause concern? Sleep specialists define "clinical" sleep apnea (sleep apnea that needs medical attention) in the following terms:

- An apnea event is when breathing stops for more than 10 seconds.
- A hypopnea event is a partial apnea in which airflow in and out of the lungs is reduced for 10 seconds or more.
- A person is considered to have clinical sleep apnea if she has more than five apnea or hypopnea events per hour.

This definition determines whether the person has sleep apnea, but it tells only part of the story.

The next question is "How severe is the sleep apnea?" That is, how sick is this person? The sleep specialist needs to answer this question to decide on the appropriate treatment.

Sleep specialists use several "yardsticks" to determine the severity of a person's sleep apnea. The simplest measure, now somewhat outdated, is called the Apnea Index. This is just the number of apnea events per hour of sleep: a person who has 30 apnea events per hour of sleep would have an apnea index of 30.

Another measurement is the total number of apnea events during an entire night. As an example, 250 apneas in an 8-hour night would not be unusual for a person with moderately serious sleep apnea.

A more accurate measure than the Apnea Index is the *Apnea-plus-Hypopnea Index* (AHI), also called the *Respiratory Disturbance Index* (RDI). The AHI (or RDI) expresses the total number of apneas plus hypopneas. The combined totals are a better measure of the severity of sleep apnea because apneas and hypopneas are equally important in causing the symptoms of sleep apnea.

Even the AHI may not give the full picture of sleep apnea severity. Another important indicator is oxygen saturation—the amount of oxygen present in the blood. Some people, despite a fairly small number of apnea events, may still be quite sick because of a very low oxygen saturation level. So the measurement of oxygen saturation is an important part of the total sleep apnea picture. Oxygen saturation is measured as a percentage. Normal is about 95 percent, and it decreases slightly as we get older. In people with sleep apnea, a blood oxygen content of approximately 80 percent during sleep is fairly common. Levels below 70 percent are considered critically low because of the high probability of irregular heart rhythm at lower blood oxygen levels.

Recently, another indicator has been proposed, the *respiratory-arousal index* (RAI). This is the total number of arousals per hour of sleep from apneas, hypopneas, and all other sleep-disordered breathing events combined.

A further aspect of the severity of sleep apnea and the need for treatment is the question of daytime sleepiness: Is sleepiness interfering with the person's life? Some people are more sensitive to sleepiness than others, and alertness is extremely critical in some occupations (for example, airplane pilot, school bus driver). The results of the multiple sleep latency test (MSLT), described earlier, give a good measurement of a person's tendency to fall asleep during the day.

Who Needs Treatment?

After your sleep test, in a follow-up visit or phone call, your sleep specialist will review your sleep test results with you: AHI, oxygen saturation record, MSLT. These data and consideration of your overall health will help the sleep specialist decide whether your sleep apnea is serious enough to need treatment.

People usually need immediate treatment if their excessive drowsiness interferes with such daily activities as driving, if it creates job hazards, if they have heart failure related to sleep apnea, or if they have very low oxygen saturation during the night. People who constantly feel tired or who have worsening high blood pressure, heart arrhythmias related to sleep apnea, badly disrupted sleep, or an AHI of more than 20 also usually need treatment.

If a person's symptoms are less severe, or the results of the sleep study show mild sleep apnea, the sleep specialist needs to carefully consider the whole picture before deciding whether to recommend treatment and, if so, how aggressive the treatment should be. See Chapter 10 for treatment of sleep apnea.

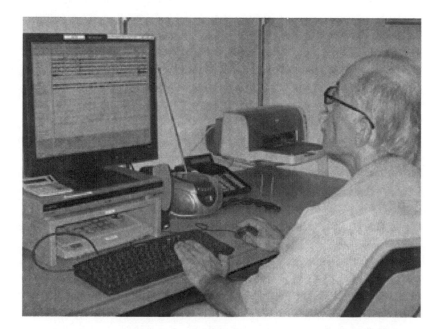

A sleep technologist reads and evaluates the electronic recording from a sleep study.

◆ Summary

- Sleep testing involves sleeping for a night at a sleep center while a device called a polysomnograph electronically records your sleep.
- You may also be asked to spend part of the next day at the sleep center for a Multiple Sleep Latency Test (MSLT).
- From the results of these tests, the sleep specialist will:
  - Decide whether you have sleep apnea; and, if so,
  - Determine how severe it is; and
  - Rule out other disorders that might accompany the sleep apnea.

Treating Sleep Apnea

- Continuous positive airway pressure (CPAP) is the treatment of choice for most people with obstructive sleep apnea. It is nearly 100 percent effective when used every night.
- Surgery should be considered as the last treatment option. There are situations where your sleep specialist and the surgeon will agree that surgery is your best first option but these are the exception.
  - The best treatment is the most conservative treatment that will work for you.
  - Nonsurgical treatments are more conservative than surgery, and may work better.
  - Get a second opinion from a sleep specialist before having surgery for sleep apnea.
- Have a sleep study before and after treatment, for comparison, to verify whether the treatment has successfully eliminated your sleep apnea.

CASE STUDY

Mr. Kennedy had a complete sleep test at an accredited sleep center. The test results showed that he had more than 250 apnea events during the night while his sleep was being recorded. His sleep specialist told him that he had moderately severe obstructive sleep apnea with a minor central apnea component, as well as cardiac arrhythmia. The specialist recommended that he undergo treatment.

At this point, Mr. Kennedy had answers to the first two questions on the pathway to successful treatment of sleep apnea:

1. Is his condition actually sleep apnea, and does he have any other conditions that will have a bearing on successful treatment?

2. What kind of sleep apnea is it (central, obstructive, or mixed), and how severe is it? (The answer to this question is important because it determines the kind of treatment.)

Finally comes the third and crucial question:

3. What is the best treatment for Mr. Kennedy's type of sleep apnea?

Choose the Right Treatment

The best treatment for anyone is the most conservative treatment that will succeed in his particular situation.

What is the most conservative treatment that will work for you? This is a complex and individual question that should be explored carefully by you, your sleep specialist, and perhaps your family doctor. The treatment should be chosen on the basis of the kind of apnea, how severe it is, and your overall health. Your sleep specialist can describe the various treatments that may work best for you and can tell you which ones are the most conservative.

What do we mean by most conservative? This means the treatment that carries the lowest risk for you.

Keep in mind that different doctors may have different treatment recommendations. Every doctor has conscious and unconscious biases in favor of certain forms of treatment. This is a natural result of his or her training, specialization, and personal experience. For example, a surgeon is more likely than an internist to believe that surgery is the best option; an internist might lean toward nonsurgical treatment.

Your job is to take these possible biases into account as you and your doctors weigh the risks and benefits and choose the most appropriate treatment for you.

CPAP Is the Right Treatment for Most People with Sleep Apnea

CPAP (continuous positive airway pressure) is the best treatment for most people with sleep apnea. CPAP completely eliminates sleep apnea, and by doing so it removes the serious risks of cardiovascular and heart disease that result from untreated sleep apnea. CPAP also improves the person's sleep, energy levels, and ability to enjoy life, so that it is possible to resume activities and career goals that have been restricted by the fatigue and exhaustion of untreated sleep apnea.

CPAP is the most conservative treatment: in the future, if other treatments are tried and turn out to be effective, CPAP can be stopped. This is a big advantage over irreversible treatments such as surgery.

CPAP is discussed in greater detail later in this chapter.

When Someone Mentions Surgery

At the first mention of surgery to treat sleep apnea, remember that:

- The best treatment is the most conservative one that works.
- The best treatment for sleep apnea, for most people, is CPAP.
- All surgery carries risk and you need to understand clearly what those risks are in your particular health situation.

Then read the section on surgery later in this chapter.

Does Insurance Pay for Sleep Apnea Treatment?

You will want to contact your insurance provider when you begin to consider treatment for sleep apnea. Ask which treatments they will pay for and exactly what that coverage includes. Most insurance providers now pay for the most common treatments for sleep apnea if the treatment is prescribed by a sleep specialist. However, some surgical procedures may not be covered.

Who Treats Sleep Apnea?

Where your treatment will be carried out will depend both on your sleep center, the size of its staff and the emphasis of its programs, and on the particular treatment. Some sleep centers provide both testing and treatment of sleep apnea, some do only sleep testing, and some fall in between these two extremes, doing some types of treatment in-house but referring patients elsewhere for others. See Chapters 16 through 18 for more information on how to obtain the health care services you need.

In any case, you can expect the sleep specialist and sleep staff to work with you and your family to plan your treatment and to recommend a treatment specialist. Your family doctor may be brought into the process at this stage.

Your sleep doctor may begin by suggesting a number of treatments that you can carry out on your own (stop smoking, lose weight, and so on). To help you with these, the sleep center may refer you to a nutritional counselor, a smokers' support group, or other such organized programs.

If surgery is an option for you, and your sleep center does not perform surgery, the center will probably suggest or recommend surgeons and other specialists with whom its staff members work frequently, and these physicians will be brought into the picture to help plan your treatment.

If your sleep center has surgeons and other specialists on the staff who can treat you there, you may still want to talk with an outside physician, preferably one with some familiarity with sleep disorders, for a second opinion before you agree to surgery.

If your treatment involves medications, the sleep center may prefer to start you on the medication and then have your family physician take over the follow-up care and monitor your progress.

The most common treatment involves the use of a breathing device. The device may be supplied through the sleep center, or the center may arrange for a homecare or medical equipment company to supply the equipment.

The First Step in Treatment: Eliminate the Obvious

The first step in treating sleep apnea is to eliminate anything that is aggravating your problem. This may improve your symptoms enough that you can avoid more complicated forms of treatment. The following can all make your sleep apnea worse:

- Alcohol, especially in the evening (even a single glass of wine with dinner), can increase the number of apnea events and decrease the level of oxygen in the blood during the night. A person with sleep apnea should avoid alcohol in the evening.
- Smoking decreases the amount of oxygen in the blood. It also causes swelling of the lining of the airway, which contributes to obstructive apnea. People with sleep apnea would be wise to stop smoking.
- Allergies and respiratory infections also cause swelling and obstruction of the airway. Treatment of allergies and upper airway infections can diminish the symptoms of obstructive sleep apnea.
- Evening medications, such as tranquilizers and short-acting beta blockers, sometimes can worsen sleep apnea. The sleep specialist may want to consult the physician who prescribed the medication to see whether a change in prescription or in medication schedule can help eliminate sleep apnea symptoms (see Appendix for list of medications that affect sleep).
- Obesity contributes greatly to obstructive sleep apnea, and weight loss can help or even eliminate sleep apnea. Weight loss is discussed in detail later in this chapter and in Chapter 11.
- Shift work. Anything that interferes with the amount and quality of sleep (as shift work does) can worsen sleep apnea symptoms. Ask your sleep specialist for information on how to improve your sleep while on shift work. You may even want to consider changing to a job that does not require rotating shifts.

Some of these aggravating factors involve lifestyles and habits that are difficult to change or to give up. Often people have the best results if they are enrolled in an organized program to help them eliminate the habit. If you find yourself trying to deal with a stubborn problem such as losing weight or stopping smoking, ask your sleep center to recommend a program that has been helpful for other people.

Treatments for Obstructive and Mixed Sleep Apnea

The current treatments for obstructive sleep apnea are (from most conservative to least conservative) change of sleeping position, weight loss, breathing devices, oral devices, drugs, and surgery.

Mixed apnea generally is treated by first treating the obstructive apnea component. Once the obstructive apnea is under control, the central apnea almost always ceases to be a problem.

Change in Sleep Position

People with obstructive sleep apnea generally have more severe apnea events when sleeping on their back; a few people have breathing difficulties only while lying on their back. A change in sleep position may eliminate the problem for these few people. However, there is no good evidence that this technique produces reliable results each night.

Even if sleep testing shows fewer breath-holds in a particular position, airflow may still be poor enough to cause sleep disruption. If you feel more rested on CPAP than you do simply sleeping on your side without CPAP, you have good evidence that you need more than just positional treatment.

Some people's apnea is so severe that even brief periods of apnea are life-threatening, and position training is not helpful.

Position change is helpful primarily to people who:

1. Have obstructive apnea that has been shown during a sleep study to occur only while lying on their back
2. Can reliably sleep on their side

Learning to avoid a particular sleep position is a matter of conditioning. Several sleep position monitors and alarms have been developed that alert sleepers when they roll onto their back and train them to choose a different sleep position. Two simple methods are sewing a small ball into the back of the pajamas or wearing to bed a small rucksack containing a bulky object that will make you lie on your side. People usually need a couple of weeks of practice before a new sleep position becomes a habit, and they may need to "retrain" themselves periodically.

Weight Loss

Who Can Be Helped by Weight Loss?

Weight loss can be effective for people with the Pickwickian syndrome (see Chapter 11 and some other overweight heavy snorers:

1. Whose apnea is associated primarily with their weight gain rather than with an anatomical obstruction of the airway (such as stuffy nose, large tonsils)
2. Whose life is not in immediate danger from the effects of sleep apnea, such as sleepiness or heart disease (see Chapter 2)

The people who are most likely to be successful at weight loss are overweight apnea sufferers who are highly motivated to improve their health and lifestyle.

Why Does Weight Loss Work?

When it is effective, weight loss works for at least two reasons- there are others that are under investigation. It relieves the abnormal loading on the abdomen that can interfere with breathing reflexes and it reduces the fatty deposits in the throat tissue that contribute to the development of obstructive apnea. However, weight loss is only effective if:

1. Sufficient weight is lost
2. The weight can be kept off permanently

Insufficient weight loss and weight regained are the two main reasons for failure of this treatment when it does fail. In fact, there may be a kind of weight "threshold" above which extra weight causes apnea symptoms and below which the symptoms are relieved. According to this theory, you need to reduce your weight far enough to fall below that threshold before you can expect to see some improvement in your apnea symptoms.

However, because the upper airway is soft sided and collapsible, it can be affected by factors other than weight gain—for example, a person whose small jaw crowds the airway may not see much improvement from weight loss.

Losing weight and keeping it off may be difficult or impossible for some people as long as their sleep apnea is untreated. Their fatigue, sleepiness, low energy, and reduced vigor may prevent them from being physically active enough to burn calories, build muscle, and successfully lose weight. In these cases, the combination of CPAP (discussed later) and weight loss can have dramatic results (see illustration on page 72). (For more on obesity, sleep apnea, and weight loss, see Chapter 11.)

Weight loss surgery is a radical way to lose weight. However, recent evidence suggests that untreated severe obesity defined by a BMI greater than 40 may have greater risks than having weight loss surgery. Even surgeons agree that weight loss surgery is not a conservative treatment and this topic is discussed later in the section on surgery.

CPAP and Similar Breathing Devices

CPAP and similar breathing devices are the most effective and most important treatment for sleep apnea. Breathing devices treat obstructive apnea by using air pressure as a "splint" to hold the upper airway open and keep it from collapsing during sleep. Some sleep experts believe that, in addition, the extra air pressure delivered by these devices may stimulate the person's breathing reflexes.

CPAP (pronounced "SEE-pap") is the most common breathing technology for treating sleep apnea. CPAP (continuous positive airway pressure) was developed in 1981 by Dr. Colin Sullivan and his research group at the University of Sydney Medical School in Australia (1,2). It was first used to treat sleep apnea patients in the United States in 1984.

CPAP is by far the most effective of all standard treatments, surgical or otherwise, for sleep apnea. For that reason, CPAP has become the treatment of choice at most sleep centers.

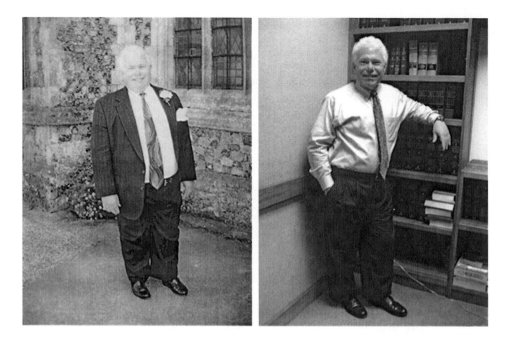

A successful weight loss patient (A) before treatment for sleep apnea and (B) 1 year later following weight management counseling and treatment for sleep apnea.

The standard CPAP system consists of a small, soft, pliable mask that is worn over the nose (usually not the mouth) at night. The mask is connected by flexible tubing to an air pump, which provides a continuous supply of slightly pressurized air through the tubing and into the nose. As soon as the CPAP wearer begins to inhale, the air pressure stabilizes his soft palate and tongue and prevents his airway from collapsing. The pressure regulator is custom set for the patient during a night in the sleep laboratory so that the CPAP delivers exactly the right pressure that the person personally needs to eliminate apnea events but no more than is necessary.

New CPAP models appear each year (see illustrations on the next page). You can see what some of the latest CPAP models and masks look like by going to the web sites of the major manufacturers of CPAP equipment and accessories:

ResMed Corp.
www.resmed.com
800-424-0737
Respironics, Inc.
www.respironics.com
800-345-6643

To read about choosing a CPAP unit and selecting a mask that fits you properly, please go to Chapters 17 and 18.

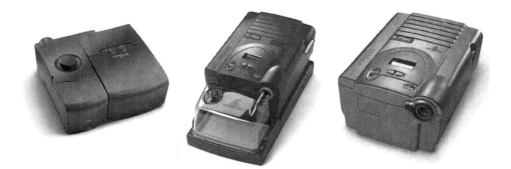

Examples of some CPAP units currently available.

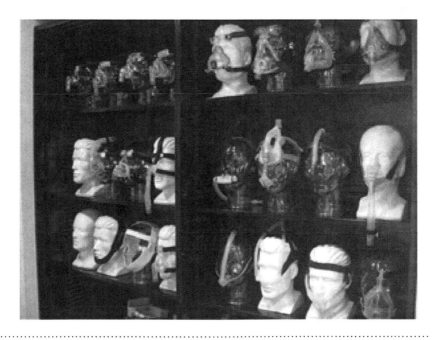

Examples of the many available sizes and styles of CPAP masks.

CPAP pressure is measured in centimeters of water (cm H_2O), in much the same way that barometric pressure is measured in millimeters of mercury (mm Hg). Typical CPAP pressure settings range from 5 to 20 cm H_2O.

Bi-level PAP (called BiPAP by the manufacturer, Respironics, Inc., see Appendix) is a refinement of CPAP. This system allows the sleep specialist to set the air pressure at two different levels: higher pressure for when the person inhales, to eliminate snoring, and lower pressure during exhaling, making it easier to exhale.

In some severe cases of obstructive sleep apnea, oxygen may be prescribed in conjunction with CPAP or bi-level PAP.

A new type of CPAP is often referred to as auto-PAP or "smart-PAP." This type of machine attempts to change pressure in response to the user's needs. The device senses the user's breathing patterns and adjusts pressure to accommodate changes in breathing that occur throughout the night. There are several manufacturers of smart-PAPs, and each one uses different breathing signals to regulate their machines. Some designs are more comfortable for the user than others, and some are more appropriate for certain types of users.

The cost of a smart-PAP is higher than for a standard CPAP. For many people with sleep apnea, the advantages probably would not justify the extra cost, nor would most insurance or health plans pay for the extra "bells and whistles" of a smart-PAP unless one is specifically prescribed. However dual- and variable-pressure systems are now the prescribed treatment of choice for more severe sleep apnea patients, and insurance usually will pay the extra cost if the sleep specialist specifically prescribes one.

The technology in this field is changing rapidly. If you are a candidate for CPAP, talk with the staff at your sleep center and with a homecare representative about the various versions of breathing devices that are available. You may want to test more than one and decide which one suits you best. See Chapter 17 for more on choosing a CPAP.

Who Can Benefit from Using CPAP?

CPAP can produce a virtual "miracle" cure in people who have not slept and breathed normally in years and are extremely ill from the long-term cardiac and respiratory effects of sleep apnea. There are probably more than 3,500,000 people in the United States using CPAP today, with the numbers growing by the tens of thousands each year. However, many people find that adapting to the use of CPAP is a challenge and requires patience and persistence.

Treatment with CPAP should be started and evaluated in the sleep center during an overnight sleep study. This allows the sleep technician to adjust the pressure correctly, establish a baseline for monitoring the effectiveness of the treatment, and avoid inappropriate or ineffectual use of CPAP. In time, CPAPs may be able to accomplish this process accurately in the patient's home. However, that time has not yet arrived.

Getting Used to CPAP

The use of CPAP requires motivation and perseverance. A few minutes are needed before going to bed each night (just like for brushing teeth) to wash the face so the skin is clean and will not be irritated by the mask, and a few more minutes every morning to wash the mask. Once CPAP is familiar, it becomes part of the bedtime routine. One needs to make a commitment to use the system each night for reasons of better health and longer life. See Chapters 17 and 18 for more on using CPAP.

CPAP users generally are willing to put up with the inconvenience once they experience the results. In one follow-up study of 20 CPAP users after about a year, 16 were still using their CPAP all night, every night (3). Such a high degree of compliance with the treatment reflects the users' enthusiasm for its effectiveness.

A high degree of compliance usually also means that the sleep disorders center has a policy of conscientious follow-up care to help new CPAP patients with problems and questions that may arise.

The main drawbacks of CPAP are related to the notion that CPAP will be cumbersome or inconvenient. Also, it may have a tendency to cause nasal irritation in some people. Some people can get used to wearing the mask in just one or two nights; others may take several weeks. The air pump motor makes a fanlike sound rather like "white noise" that a few CPAP users find annoying. Newer CPAP machines have gotten so quiet that patients who wake up in the night sometimes find that they cannot hear their CPAP machine at all and, until they are accustomed to it, they feel they need to check to be sure it is still working. Most people do not object to the sound or the presence of CPAP, and their bedmates generally prefer CPAP over snoring.

When used all night, every night, CPAP provides positive results that are close to an instant cure. After beginning to use CPAP, most people report that within days they feel better than they have felt in many years. They report sleeping better, feeling rested in the morning and alert during the day, and having the energy to do the things they have been longing to do.

When regular CPAP users stop using it for a night—for example, during a power failure—they generally are eager to return to CPAP because the apneas and their symptoms promptly return. In fact, after using CPAP and then sleeping without it, many people report that they had never been so aware of the choking they experienced with each apnea event. Now if they sleep without CPAP, they dream that heavy weights have been placed on their chest or they awaken feeling suffocated, so they are not often tempted to give up their CPAP.

Please read Chapter 17 before you purchase a CPAP and Chapter 18 for suggestions on sleeping comfortably with a CPAP.

What Are the Long-Term Effects of Using CPAP?

Since the introduction of CPAP in the 1980s sleep scientists have been watching carefully for any unfavorable long-term effects. By now thousands of people have been using CPAP for more than 20 years, and no serious negative consequences have been reported in the medical literature. Of course, no one can guarantee the safety of sleeping for 30 or 40 years under slightly higher air pressure, but so far the medical literature suggests that the long-term risks from sleep apnea are much more dangerous than any potential long-term risks from using CPAP.

How Much Do CPAP Devices Cost?

CPAP systems can be obtained by rental or purchase. It is a good idea to begin by renting a system for 2 or 3 months, seeing how you do with it, and perhaps trying a couple of different models. Costs vary around the country. Currently, CPAP unit rentals cost approximately $250 to $350 per month, and the purchase price is in the neighborhood of $1,500 to $3,000. You may have to purchase the mask and tubing separately (about $200). The mask material tends to absorb oil from the skin and become stiff, so masks require periodic replacement. Silicone masks may last up to 18 months. A heated humidifier can cost $500, an unheated one closer to $100.

Your health insurance may cover most, if not all, of the costs of CPAP, both rental and purchase. Talk to your insurance company representative to find out which equipment and supplies they will cover (see Chapter 17 for more on selecting a CPAP).

How Can You Obtain a CPAP Unit?

You must have a doctor's prescription to obtain a CPAP machine. Your sleep center personnel can put you in touch with a homecare company that will supply you with a CPAP system. The homecare company representative will teach you how to operate your CPAP unit. They should provide same-day service in case of breakdown. (See Chapters 17 and 18 on homecare companies.)

Some sleep centers rent or sell CPAP systems directly. However, most do not have the desire or the staff that this requires.

Oral Devices for Treating Sleep Apnea

A number of oral devices have been designed for treating sleep apnea, with the objective of holding the lower jaw, the tongue, or both in a forward position during sleep, hoping to make the upper airway less likely to collapse. These devices are likely to work best for people whose obstructive apnea originates primarily in the lower pharynx (throat) from the position of their tongue or lower jaw in relation to their airway.

Jaw Retainers (Mandibular Advancement Devices, or MADs)

Jaw retainers are dental appliances that hold the lower jaw forward (4,5). We will call them MADs (mandibular advancement devices), although they are also called mandibular repositioning devices (MRDs), anterior mandibular positioners (AMPs), or oral airway dilators (OADs).

MADs look like the bite plates or retainers that sometimes are prescribed by orthodontists. They are made of dental acrylic and may have metal loops over several teeth to hold the device in place (see illustration on page 77). Many different manufacturers have designed their own MAD versions. Some models are adjustable for easy selection of the best forward position for the lower jaw. Most MADs must be custom fitted.

Definitive studies to pinpoint who will benefit from a jaw retainer or which devices work best have not been completed. Studies of mandibular appliances in sleep apnea patients have used small numbers of patients and different definitions of "success." So far, these limited clinical trials suggest that mandibular devices are about 50 percent effective. That is, about half of patients who try them still have serious enough sleep apnea symptoms that they need additional treatment. The adjustable models may be more practical than models that are not adjustable. It is unlikely that any one design will work equally well for all patients.

For these and other reasons, people who are considering an oral appliance would be wise to locate a dentist who is experienced in using these devices for the treatment

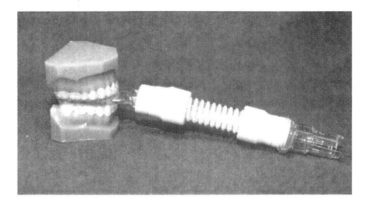

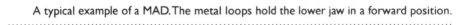

A typical example of a MAD. The metal loops hold the lower jaw in a forward position.

of sleep apnea and who works in cooperation with a sleep specialist. The sleep specialist (not the dentist) should make the diagnosis of obstructive sleep apnea and should measure the effectiveness of the dental device after the dentist has fit the patient with it. You can locate a dentist near you who has been trained in this field by contacting the Academy of Dental Sleep Medicine (see Appendix).

Who Can Benefit from Using a MAD?   The manufacturers of MADs and some experimenters who have studied patients using them have reported some good results, especially in patients who have mild to moderate apnea (5–8).

Because MADs focus their treatment on the lower jaw and/or tongue, people with a smallish lower jaw that is set somewhat far back (called by orthodontists a class II occlusion) are likely to have the best results.

MADs also have been used successfully in children born with irregularly formed jaws who have difficulty with obstructive apnea.

Three-quarters of people with sleep apnea have airway obstructions in more than one place. People whose obstructive apnea results mostly from nasal problems or from the upper pharynx (large tonsils, adenoids, soft palate, uvula) are not likely to be treated successfully with an MAD and will need further treatment. In fact, you must be able to breathe through your nose to use the retainer; a person with a nasal obstruction or a stuffy nose from an allergy or a cold will be unable to wear one. Even some people who seem likely candidates for MADs continue to have apnea events, as shown by heavy snoring. Also, it is necessary to have enough teeth to be able to hold an appliance in place.

One group of people who may want to try an MAD are those who have been unable to use CPAP despite a wholehearted effort. However, if a nasal obstruction is preventing you from successfully using CPAP, you will also be unable to use an oral appliance unless you can eliminate the nasal obstruction by surgery or medication.

There may be a place for occasional use of an MAD, even if it is only partially effective, for example:

1. When CPAP is unavailable (backpacking, primitive travel)
2. When the device allows the patient to use a lower CPAP pressure
3. When screening patients for mandibular advancement surgery (to simulate the possible results of surgery)

Objective studies of the benefit in these situations are not yet available.

Getting Used to a MAD.   It may take from several nights to several weeks to get completely accustomed to wearing a MAD. Excess saliva will probably be an early side effect. Any foreign object in the mouth, such as a retainer, causes the production of excess saliva at first, but this generally tapers off after a night or two. However, it may take as long as 2 or 3 weeks for jaw muscles and other muscles to become accustomed to wearing a MAD. You may need to wear it at least that long to carry out a fair trial and decide whether it is effective.

A disadvantage of the MAD is that you cannot rent one to try it out. One "do-it-yourself" brand, which is available by prescription, can be adapted to fit by warming it in hot water. It works well enough to offer some idea of effectiveness, but it is not very durable. Otherwise, you will not know whether a MAD works for you until you have paid to have one made. If it does work, you will be delighted. A MAD is less restrictive of movement, much smaller, less expensive, and more convenient to deal with than a breathing device. If it does not work, other options are available.

How Much Do MADs Cost?   MADs are less expensive than CPAP units, but still surprisingly costly. The do-it-yourself brand costs about $25. Some sleep centers have trained technicians who can fit an adjustable model for $300 to $400. Some manufacturers charge as much as $600 for a custom-fitted appliance, and with the dentist's markup it may cost you more than $1,000. That is approximately twice the cost of an ordinary orthodontic retainer and does not include the cost of having your orthodontist or dentist take jaw impressions, or the cost of additional visits to check or adjust the fit of the appliance. This can add another several hundred dollars to the cost. Check with your insurance company in advance to see if they will cover part or all of these costs.

Should You Try a MAD?   If you and your sleep specialist think you are a likely candidate for success with an MAD, here are some questions to answer:

1. Have you had a sleep study to measure the baseline of your sleep apnea before treatment?
2. Is your sleep apnea mild?
3. If your sleep apnea is moderate to severe, have you tried CPAP (a more effective treatment)?
4. Do you have nasal obstructions that would prevent you from breathing through your nose?

5. Do you have temporomandibular joint (TMJ) syndrome or dental problems that might be aggravated by using an MAD?
6. If you have TMJ or dental problems, can your sleep specialist refer you to a dentist who is experienced in fitting oral appliances for sleep apnea?
7. Has your sleep specialist scheduled you for a follow-up sleep study while you are wearing the oral appliance to verify its effectiveness?
8. Have you added up and talked with your insurance agent about the full costs of an oral device, including fabrication, fitting, office visits for adjustments, and a follow-up sleep test? Do you consider this a cost-effective treatment option?

These questions are based partly on standards suggested by the American Academy of Sleep Medicine for the use of oral appliances (9).

Is Your MAD Really Working?   Soon after you become accustomed to using an MAD, you should return to the sleep center for a follow-up sleep study to determine whether the appliance is effectively eliminating your apnea. The sleep study must assess whether the MAD works both when you are sleeping on your back and when you are sleeping on your side.

An important disadvantage of MADs is that their effectiveness tends to decrease over a period of a year or two (10). Consequently, you should consult your sleep specialist about when to schedule a follow-up sleep study to make sure your MAD is still eliminating your sleep apnea.

Other Oral Appliances

The Tongue-Retaining Device.   The tongue-retaining device (TRD) is made of soft plastic and consists of a tongue-sized suction cup that is supposed to pull the tongue forward and hold it in that position. It is gripped by the teeth and held in place during sleep (11,12).

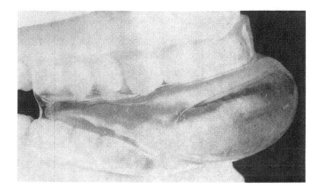

A Samelson-type TRD. The tongue is drawn forward into the bubble and held by suction.

Many people who have used the TRD in experiments have found it moderately uncomfortable to wear. For this reason, it was worn only half the night in some experiments. Despite its drawbacks, the TRD was found to decrease the number of apnea events by approximately 50 percent. This means that the TRD could be about as effective as uvulopalatopharyngoplasty (UPPP), a type of surgery described later.

The TRD has not excited a lot of enthusiasm in the sleep research community, and so far it has not become widely used or available. Part of the reason for this probably is that the TRD apparently is useful only to a small group of obstructive apnea patients.

The people who are most likely to be helped by a TRD are those who are not obese, have no nasal obstructions, and have only mild to moderate apnea that is strongly influenced by sleeping position—that is, the apnea is much worse when sleeping on the back than when sleeping on the side (12). For this group of people, apnea apparently is strongly affected by tongue position; therefore, holding the tongue forward with the TRD might be helpful. In some cases, more severe apnea has been controlled with the use of a TRD.

Oral Positive Airway Pressure Appliance. The oral positive airway pressure (OPAP) appliance treats obstructive sleep apnea with a mouthpiece instead of a nose mask. It consists of a small mouthpiece that can be worn either by itself or connected to CPAP tubing and a CPAP machine. By itself, the OPAP appliance can be used like a jaw retainer to hold the lower jaw in a forward position if desired. Attached to a CPAP unit, it holds the airway open with air pressure, just like a CPAP unit (13).

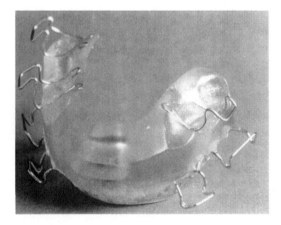

An OPAP appliance.

Who Can Be Helped by an OPAP Appliance? The OPAP appliance may be an alternative for people with mild to severe obstructive sleep apnea who would otherwise be using a standard CPAP mask, or have had difficulty using CPAP, or have had unsuccessful surgery for obstructive sleep apnea. Worn by itself, the OPAP appliance might be considered an alternative dental appliance to treat obstructive sleep apnea. The advantage of the OPAP appliance is that it bypasses the nose, where many people have nasal obstructions that make CPAP use difficult. It also avoids the mask-fitting issues of CPAP and the skin irritation that some people experience from wearing the CPAP mask against the face. The OPAP appliance does not require headgear, so it may be more comfortable, and it eliminates the "bad hair day" that can greet a person in the morning after wearing CPAP headgear all night.

What Are the Drawbacks of OPAP?   OPAP is so new that very few patients have had a chance to try it. Excessive production of saliva is likely the most obvious drawback. Long-term effects are not yet available. Questions remain about how OPAP affects the teeth and the temporomandibular joint (TMJ). People with TMJ problems should consult their dentist about using an OPAP appliance.

How Much Does an OPAPAppliance Cost?   At present, an OPAP appliance is custom fit like a dental appliance, which can be costly. The cost will probably be in the neighborhood of $600. A less expensive, off-the-shelf model may be available in the future. If you are considering an OPAP appliance, you should contact your insurance company and ask whether they will cover the cost.

How Can You Get an OPAP Appliance?   Ask your sleep specialist whether an OPAP appliance would be appropriate for you. If so, she should be able to refer you to a dentist who is trained to fit an OPAP appliance. If not, contact the Academy of Dental Sleep Medicine (see Appendix) for the name of a dentist who is trained to treat sleep disorders and familiar with these devices.

Orthodontic Treatment to Remodel the Jaw

Orthodontists are playing an increasing role in the treatment of obstructive sleep apnea. Sleep apnea patients who have a small jaw—class II malocclusion–have a crowded, easily obstructed airway. Orthodontic treatment is able to remodel the jaw by moving teeth apart and using implants to fill the spaces (14). This treatment, alone or combined with jaw surgery (see below), may enlarge the jaw sufficiently to reduce or eliminate obstruction of the airway.

Orthodontists have begun to recognize the risk of inviting obstructive sleep apnea in the future by removing childhood teeth to "make room" in the jaw. The problem with this practice is that, over the years, the jaw bones tend to restructure themselves in response to the actions of chewing and movement of the tongue muscle. With fewer teeth occupying space, the jaw may end up smaller, with crowded teeth, overbite, and a crowded airway. The unintended consequence may be obstructive sleep apnea.

In the future, a more common solution to childhood's crowded jaw may turn out to be preservation of the size and architecture of the jaw rather than removal of teeth.

Drugs for Treating Obstructive Sleep Apnea

So far, drugs generally are not very effective in treating obstructive sleep apnea. However, several of the drugs that have been tried unsuccessfully as treatments for central apnea (described previously) have met with at least mixed success in obstructive apnea.

The hormone medroxyprogesterone has been found to be somewhat effective in some people with the Pickwickian syndrome (see Chapter 11). It has been reported to improve the breathing drive, to decrease the number of apnea events, and to improve the patient's symptoms (15–17). However, some researchers have reported no improvement in apneas, so the results with this drug are conflicting (15–18).

Medroxyprogesterone has some undesirable side effects. It can cause fluid retention, nausea, and depression in some people. Because it is a sex hormone, it may cause extra hair growth and breast tenderness. It should not be used by people with blood-clotting disorders or liver disease, by pregnant women, or by people known or suspected to have genital cancer.

Protriptyline is an antidepressant that is variably effective in mild cases of sleep apnea. It is only a treatment option if the person's life is not in immediate danger from the effects of sleep apnea.

Drawbacks of protriptyline are that it decreases the amount of rapid eye movement (REM) sleep and has a high incidence of other side effects, including dry mouth, constipation (mild to intolerable), difficulty starting urine flow, and impotence (16,19). It can cause confusion, especially in elderly people. It may not be appropriate for people with arrhythmias, very high blood pressure, glaucoma, or prostate disease (17).

Oxygen alone is not an effective treatment for obstructive sleep apnea; in fact, it can make obstructive apnea worse.

Surgery for Obstructive Sleep Apnea

Surgical Risks to Consider

Surgery is the least conservative treatment for obstructive sleep apnea, and for most people it is not likely to be as effective as CPAP. It would be wise to understand the other alternatives before selecting this one. And by all means get a second opinion from a different physician before deciding on surgery.

The most conservative treatments for sleep apnea do not involve surgery. They may involve some inconvenience or perseverance, but they do not expose the patient to the risks of pain and possible complications or death that are inherent in any surgical procedure.

A conservative surgical procedure meets most or all of the following criteria:

- It is a routine procedure that has been carried out for many years rather than a new or experimental type of surgery.
- It does not involve cutting major blood vessels or nerves, dealing with major organs, or entering a body cavity.

- It normally has no serious postoperative complications.
- It can be performed by a surgeons who are experienced with this particular surgical procedure without much variation in outcome.
- It can be done safely on an outpatient basis or involves, at most, a minimal (one- or two-day) hospital stay.

Surgery has many potential pitfalls: pain, excessive loss of blood, reactions to medications, nerve or muscle damage, infection, wound breakdown, and other complications (20,21).

One of the biggest risks from surgery is general anesthesia (20). This is particularly true for a person with sleep apnea. Anesthetics depress the breathing reflexes, and a person with sleep apnea already has some degree of respiratory difficulty. Anyone with sleep apnea who is having surgery should warn the surgeon in advance that he has sleep apnea. Better yet, the person could ask the sleep specialist to consult with the surgeon. The surgeon and the anesthesiologist should both be aware that this person's breathing will need to be monitored very carefully during and immediately after surgery.

So even "simple" surgery should be considered very carefully. Surgery may be the only option that makes sense for a person who is very sick as a result of sleep apnea—it may be necessary to save his or her life. For other people who are not in immediate danger from the severe long-term effects of apnea or who may simply want to "stop snoring," the potential risks involved in some of the surgical procedures may outweigh the possible benefits.

Can Surgery Cure Sleep Apnea?

Help versus Cure?   It is important to distinguish between an attempt to *help* sleep apnea and an attempt to cure sleep apnea (that is, eliminate all disease, including the high risk of stroke, heart attack, and other cardiovascular disease caused by untreated sleep apnea). For example, patients A and B might both show a significant decrease in sleep apnea after surgery. However, patient A might have started out with mild apnea and may not need further treatment despite some remaining sleep apnea. (An example would be a person who goes from a sleepy patient with a respiratory disturbance index [AHI] of 40 before surgery to an alert patient with an AHI of 10 after surgery.) Patient B, on the other hand, might have started with more serious apnea and may still need to use CPAP after surgery. (An example would be a person whose AHI of 60 improves to 30 after surgery but who still has low blood oxygen at night, still has a high risk of cardiovascular disease, and is still drowsy.)

Results Vary Among Individuals.   The surgical procedures for sleep apnea are not equally effective for all people. For example, an early surgical procedure that was used for sleep apnea and is still being used today is uvulopalatopharyngoplasty (UPPP) (described later). As a treatment for sleep apnea, UPPP has about a 50 percent failure rate, and after 5 years, the success rate may fall to as low as 25 percent. This means that 50 percent of the people who undergo this surgery still have a significant problem with sleep apnea immediately after surgery, and the percentage of people with problems will increase with time.

Surgery for reconstructing the lower jaw (mandibular advancement and its variations) also has a fairly high nonsuccess rate but when combined simultaneously with maxillary surgery it has helped individuals with even severe sleep apnea.

There are several reasons for the failure of surgery to correct sleep apnea. One is simply inappropriate choice of treatment. There are some patients for whom it can be predicted in advance that UPPP is not likely to cure their apnea. Yet, some of these patients choose to have surgery anyway. Quite often, after a person is diagnosed with sleep apnea, she is not ready to accept the reality of having a long-term health condition, and may seize upon surgery as a hopeful "quick fix." Or the person may be referred directly to a surgeon by a family doctor who is unfamiliar with or biased against nonsurgical treatments for sleep apnea. Poor surgical candidates usually find that their sleep apnea returns after surgery and that they still need long-term treatment.

Another reason for the low success rate of surgery is the newness of treating sleep apnea with surgery. There still are not enough data to be able to predict accurately which people will be cured by a particular reconstructive procedure.

Before you choose surgery for the treatment of sleep apnea, ask your sleep specialist about the chances of success for you, and listen carefully to the answer.

To summarize, be sure you are an excellent candidate for the particular kind of surgery you are considering before you take the risk of having it. A second opinion from a qualified sleep specialist who will not be performing the surgery is strongly advised.

One final point on choosing a conservative treatment: If you are considering being treated at a medical school, you might keep in mind that medical schools may lean toward more aggressive, more experimental, less conservative treatment options. Although this is fine from the point of view of advancing medical science, you should ask yourself whether you want to risk being part of that process.

Five Categories of Surgery for Sleep Apnea

Five general types of surgery are used to treat obstructive sleep apnea:

1. Nasal surgery
2. Palate and tongue surgeries
   • UPPP (uvulopalatopharyngoplasty)
   • LAUP (laser-assisted uvulopalatoplasty for snoring)
   • Somnoplasty (radiofrequency thermal ablation)
3. Jaw surgery and other maxillofacial surgeries
4. Tracheostomy
5. Weight loss surgery

Nasal Surgery   Nasal surgery actually may refer to several different ear, nose, and throat (ENT) procedures. These can include repair of the nasal septum (the wall that separates your left and right nasal passages), turbinate surgery to remove bony obstructions, removal of polyps, surgery on the nasal sinuses, or submucous resection (removing loose tissue under the lining of the nasal passages).

Nasal surgery may be a necessary first step to allow some people to use CPAP. People with nasal obstructions may feel "claustrophobic" or suffocated while using CPAP, or they may unconsciously pull off the CPAP mask during sleep. CPAP users who have these problems should ask their sleep specialist whether nasal surgery might make them more comfortable with CPAP.

Nasal surgery may also permit a person to wear an oral appliance (mandibular advancement device) that would have been impossible before surgery. A person who has poor airflow through the nose would feel suffocated wearing an oral appliance.

By itself, nasal surgery usually is not an effective treatment for sleep apnea or snoring. Some people occasionally report a decrease in snoring after surgery on their nose, only to have the symptoms return over several months.

However, improved airflow through the nose can have a significant effect on overall airflow, and it should also be considered as part of an overall surgical approach if palate surgery (see the next section) is going to be carried out.

Palate and Tongue Surgeries UVULOPALATOPHARYNGOPLASTY. UPPP was the first and remains the most common type of surgery for sleep apnea. Under general anesthesia, a scalpel is used to remove approximately the rear third of the soft palate. The back of the soft palate is left in a streamlined shape that will be less likely to collapse during sleep.

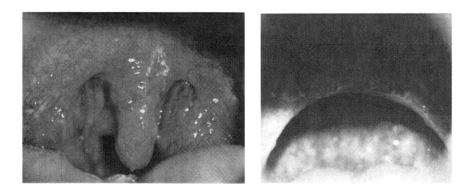

UPPP surgery: (A) Before. Notice the large tonsils and fleshy uvula. (B) After. Tonsils and uvula have been removed.

Who Can Be Helped by UPPP? Whether a person can be helped by UPPP depends on the reason for surgery and on how one defines being "helped." If the surgery is for purely "cosmetic" purposes (that is, simply to cut down on snoring) and if a sleep study has shown that the person has only snoring and not sleep apnea, UPPP stands about a

90 percent chance of being successful. The bedmate's report that snoring has disappeared after UPPP does not necessarily mean the disappearance of sleep apnea.

If the purpose of surgery is to eliminate sleep apnea completely, the chance of success is much lower and much more difficult to predict, but probably is less than 20 percent. People who are the most likely candidates for success with this type of surgery meet the following criteria:

1. They are not more than 25 percent or 30 percent over their ideal weight, and they do not gain weight after surgery (22,23).
2. They have only mild to moderate apnea, and it is all obstructive apnea.
3. Their apnea arises mostly from some obvious anatomical obstruction of the upper part of the pharynx (throat)—the soft palate or upper throat area (24,25). This includes people with enlarged tonsils or adenoids (tonsils and adenoids often are removed during UPPP); people with a very long soft palate or a large, fleshy uvula; and people with excess fleshy tissue in the throat region. The combination of abnormally large palatal tissue with large obstructive tonsils may give the best outcome- UPPP combined with tonsillectomy.

In contrast, people with very severe apnea or those whose apnea arises from places other than the area of the soft palate are not good candidates for UPPP. Those with a lower jaw that is very short or placed far back, or with a tongue that is large or is positioned fairly far back and low in the neck, or with apnea arising in the lower pharynx are less likely to be successful with UPPP (25,26).

Weight gain is an extremely important factor in the success of UPPP. Extra loading of the abdomen, which interferes with the breathing reflex, plus fatty deposits in the neck, which help obstruct the airway, can overpower any positive results that may be gained from UPPP. Therefore, people who have UPPP and then gain weight are likely to see the return of obstructive apnea (22).

Until recently, not much was known about which people could best be helped by UPPP. With the aid of cephalometry (measurement of size and placement of structures in the head using radiographs, computed tomography (CT), or magnetic resonance imaging [MRI]) and fiberoptic examination of the inside of the airway, doctors are gradually gaining more information about how to choose the most likely candidates for successful UPPP (26–30). Nevertheless, no one can accurately predict the success of UPPP.

Determining whether you are a good candidate for UPPP must be done by consulting your sleep expert and a good otolaryngologist (ENT specialist) who has experience not only with eliminating snoring but also with sleep apnea problems. The otolaryngologist should examine your throat internally. He may order a radiograph, MRI, or CT scan of your head so that he can measure the sizes and relationships between various anatomical features that cause your obstructive apnea. This will help to determine your chances of being helped by UPPP.

What Are the Drawbacks to Uvulopalatopharyngoplasty?   Compared with many surgical procedures, uvulopalatopharyngoplasty is not particularly risky. It does not involve any large arteries or nerves. It may be performed as outpatient surgery in healthy, uncomplicated cases. A hospital stay of 1 or 2 days may be necessary for some patients.

As mentioned previously, the greatest risk probably is from the anesthesia. The more narrow the airway, the greater the risk from preoperative medications, from anesthetics, and from painkillers and sedatives given immediately after the operation (20).

The reason for this increased risk is that anesthetics and some other drugs interfere with the breathing reflexes. If you have sleep apnea, you already have breathing reflexes that may not operate quite normally. This means that you are at somewhat greater than normal risk from anesthesia. This breathing abnormality, coupled with existing apnea, possible throat obstruction from postoperative swelling, and perhaps pain medication could add up to serious complications.

Pain is another consideration with UPPP. People who have had UPPP report that the pain after the operation is very severe—more painful than expected (for example, more painful than a tonsillectomy). Severe pain can last as long as a week.

All patients report difficulty with swallowing after surgery. The removal of the uvula at the back of the mouth cavity makes it easier for food or liquid in the mouth to be pushed up into the back of the nasal cavity during swallowing. This is a common problem for the first 2 weeks after surgery, but it should correct itself with time, particularly if the surgeon is skilled and experienced with the procedure. A few people continue to have swallowing problems. However, most who do have a little difficulty swallowing find that they overcome the problem with some practice and if they eat properly (20,23).

There have been reports of airway obstruction becoming worse or more difficult to treat with CPAP following UPPP.

Why Have Uvulopalatopharyngoplasty If the Odds Are Poor? Even if you have only a 50/50 chance of being helped enough not to require further treatment, you may prefer taking that chance in the hope of avoiding other treatments, such as CPAP, oral appliances, or other surgeries.

UPPP has a very low risk when performed on patients who have been carefully tested at a good sleep center, and when the surgery is performed by an experienced ENT surgeon. For example, currently we are not aware of a surgical fatality or a serious complication from this surgery at the Swedish[sws7] Medical Center.

How Can You Arrange for Uvulopalatopharyngoplasty? It is not wise to have UPPP as a treatment for sleep apnea until you have been thoroughly examined by a physician who understands the causes of sleep apnea and knows how to weigh the benefits against the risks in your particular case. The sleep specialist, in turn, can refer you to a surgeon who is experienced with UPPP if you appear to be a good candidate for successful treatment by this procedure.

LASER SURGERY TO TREAT SNORING. Laser-assisted uvulopalatoplasty (LAUP) is a technique for surgery on the soft palate that has been promoted as a harmless way to eliminate simple snoring. However, snoring is a symptom of sleep apnea, and in definitive studies LAUP has not been shown to be an effective treatment for sleep apnea (31,32).

The distinction between simple snoring and sleep apnea is not always clear. People who appear to have "simple snoring" frequently turn out to have significant sleep apnea (31). LAUP surgeons often try to screen out those patients with a questionnaire on snoring. However, questionnaires cannot accurately diagnose sleep apnea and tend to underestimate it. Consequently, many patients with undiagnosed sleep apnea have had LAUP surgery and have been left with a serious underlying disorder. To avoid unnecessary, possibly harmful LAUP surgery, people who snore should first be evaluated by a sleep specialist to rule out sleep apnea. LAUP should be considered only after sleep apnea has been ruled out.

LAUP has been promoted as a substitute for conventional palate surgery (that is, UPPP, as described previously). Patients whose sleep and ENT specialists consider them good candidates for UPPP for treatment of snoring may want to consider LAUP for this purpose, but not to treat sleep apnea.

What Is LAUP?   LAUP involves several lengthwise laser "cuts" making a V-shaped pattern on the soft palate. Several sessions usually are needed. The laser cauterizes ("cooks") the tissue, leaving narrow scars that stiffen the soft palate and presumably diminish the vibration that causes snoring.

Does LAUP Eliminate Snoring?   Proponents claim that it does in 80 percent to 90 percent of cases, but there are reports that snoring may return within 2 years after surgery.[33]

How Does LAUP Compare with Conventional UPPP?   LAUP is less risky—it involves less time, less bleeding, less tissue removal, no general anesthetic, and no hospitalization. It is somewhat less expensive (expect charges of approximately $1,600 for the surgeon, plus an additional fee for the surgical facility). Conventional UPPP involves a general anesthetic; possibly a hospital stay; significant pain; and risks from bleeding, infection, and general anesthetic. UPPP may cost up to $3,000.

Please read the previous sections in this chapter on choosing surgery in general and on choosing UPPP.

Can LAUP Cure Sleep Apnea?   No, it cannot, according to published analyses (31). LAUP may be helpful as an adjunct treatment for mild to moderate apnea, with approximately 50 percent of patients obtaining 50 percent or better improvement. Careful examination of the airway may identify people who are likely to have poor results. These include patients with a large tongue and a small palate.

The main danger from LAUP is that people who have a potentially fatal disorder, sleep apnea, may have LAUP under the mistaken impression that the surgery will cure them. Sleep apnea is more than snoring (see Chapter 7, "What Causes Sleep Apnea?").

The American Academy of Sleep Medicine's standards of practice for LAUP recommend that patients be evaluated by a sleep specialist before having LAUP. People with sleep apnea should have a follow-up sleep study after surgery to determine whether the sleep apnea has been eliminated (32).

SOMNOPLASTY (RADIOFREQUENCY SURGICAL ABLATION) Somnoplasty is another newer technique. It uses radio-frequency energy to shrink the bulk of soft tissue. In 1998, the U.S. Food and Drug Administration (FDA) approved Somnoplasty on the upper airway (for example, soft palate and base of tongue) for treatment of sleep apnea.

Like LAUP, Somnoplasty is being promoted to the general public as a simple solution for the common, desperately annoying problem of snoring. As with LAUP, patients run the risk of bypassing an important medical issue—undiagnosed sleep apnea. Like LAUP, Somnoplasty by itself does not appear to be an effective treatment for moderate to severe sleep apnea. It may be helpful in milder cases, perhaps in combination with other treatments such as CPAP, weight loss, or an oral appliance. Definitive controlled studies on Somnoplasty have not yet been published.

How Does Somnoplasty Work? Somnoplasty uses high-frequency radio waves to destroy cells by heating them and causing the formation of a scar. The scar shrinks and reduces the bulk of the tissue. A crude version of this technology has been used for years in surgery to cauterize bleeding capillaries and to eliminate small tumors. In the case of Somnoplasty, a much lower level of energy is used.

The procedure is performed in the doctor's office. The operator anesthetizes the area and then inserts a thin electrode into the tissue. The electrode emits radio-frequency energy that creates a lesion; basically the energy "cooks" a small area of tissue. Each lesion takes 3 to 6 minutes to create, and several lesions usually are made during a single session.

Swelling occurs within the few days after the surgical session, and scar tissue replaces the lesions within a couple of weeks. The scarring shrinks the area and decreases the bulk of the tissue. The amount of the decrease depends on the amount of scarring produced (34).

Two to four surgical sessions are reported to be needed for best results, with 8 weeks for healing between sessions.

What Are the Risks from Somnoplasty? Because Somnoplasty requires only a local rather than a general anesthetic, it may involve fewer surgical risks than scalpel surgery. No significant side effects had been reported after 1 year of experience with Somnoplasty. Long-term results are not yet known.

Swelling occurs after the surgery, which can be risky for sleep apnea patients who have difficulty keeping their airway open. Patients should sleep at a 45-degree angle after surgery while they still have some swelling.

A risk that Somnoplasty shares with LAUP is that it silences the major warning sign of sleep apnea by eliminating snoring, and patients can be left to unknowingly suffer the long-term effects of an undiagnosed, potentially harmful disorder.

Another potential risk with Somnoplasty relates to the training and experience of the person performing the operation. If you are considering Somnoplasty, you would be wise to ask about the medical qualifications of the individual who will be performing the actual procedure.

Can Palate Somnoplasty Effectively Treat Sleep Apnea?   In palate surgery by Somnoplasty, a series of lesions are created in the soft palate over the course of three or four surgical sessions, with the goal of shrinking and tightening the palate.

The FDA has approved the use of Somnoplasty on the upper airway (palate, tongue) as a treatment for sleep apnea. However, it is unlikely to be more effective than LAUP or UPPP for apnea because it affects the same tissue. Long-term results are not yet available.

A reputable Somnoplasty practitioner will ask you whether you have symptoms of sleep apnea, counsel you about its possible dangers, and refer you for appropriate sleep testing. If this does not happen, and if you have underlying sleep apnea, do not count on a cure from Somnoplasty.

It is extremely important to return to your sleep specialist and have a sleep study following Somnoplasty to find out whether your sleep apnea has been eliminated even if you feel that it has.

Can Palate Somnoplasty Eliminate Snoring?   Reports suggest that it can decrease or eliminate snoring about as well as LAUP. Long-term results are not yet available.

Tongue Reduction by Somnoplasty.   In tongue reduction by Somnoplasty (35), the goal is to decrease the bulk of the tongue so it does not obstruct the throat. In the past, a scalpel or laser was used to remove a notch of tissue at the back of the tongue, sometimes along with some tonsillar tissue that is located at the base of the tongue (36). Because Somnoplasty is such a new technique, no one knows whether this type of surgery on the tongue will be more or less effective than the laser method, so results are difficult to predict. The success of tongue reduction surgery in treating apnea also is difficult to predict. Two groups of surgeons reported the results of laser tongue surgery on 24 patients who had already had unsuccessful UPPP surgery (36,37). Following laser tongue surgery, fewer than half of the procedures were considered "successful," and those patients still had an average RDI above 10 and blood oxygen levels below 90, which means that many of them would still end up on CPAP. Tongue Somnoplasty is still an experimental procedure, but shows some promise as a treatment for obstructive sleep apnea.

How Does Somnoplasty Compare with LAUP and Conventional UPPP?   Somnoplasty is less risky than UPPP, involving less bleeding, no hospitalization, and no general anesthetic. According to one published report, Somnoplasty is less painful than LAUP during recovery. The cost of Somnoplasty currently is $1,600 to $2,000 and usually is not paid for by insurance if it is performed for primary snoring alone.

PILLAR PROCEDURE.   The Pillar procedure is a new surgical procedure using plastic implants to stiffen the soft palate. It appears to be moderately successful at decreasing snoring. Currently, very few sleep apnea patients have had this surgery. Early results show a slight improvement in the Apnea-Hypopnea Index (38,39). No long-term results are available. The verdict on the effectiveness of the Pillar procedure in treating sleep apnea will have to wait until more patients have had the procedure and further data on both short term and long term results are available.

Jaw Surgery and Other Maxillofacial Surgeries Maxillofacial surgery is surgery on the mandible (lower jaw), the maxilla (upper jaw), and the other bones and tissue of the face. Head and neck surgery involves the other parts of the head, face, and airway, and is performed by otolaryngologists, or ENTs. Surgeries have a 20-year history of use as a treatment for sleep apnea, but it is still difficult to predict which sleep apnea patients are most likely to have their sleep apnea eliminated by this type of surgery. These surgeries include individually or in combination:

- Mandibular advancement—moves the lower jaw forward
- Midface advancement—moves the maxilla (upper jaw) forward
- Hyoid surgery—repositions the base of the tongue

Jaw surgery and other maxillofacial surgeries for treating sleep apnea actually include half a dozen possible surgical procedures and many variations. All are aimed at eliminating obstructions in the airway that lies behind the lower jaw.

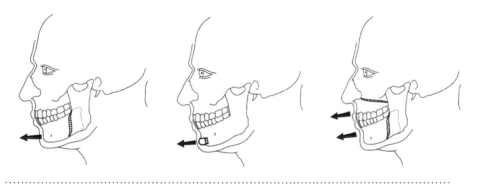

Examples of mandibular and maxillofacial surgeries that have been tried for treating obstructive sleep apnea: (A) and (B), two ways of pulling the lower jaw and the base of the tongue forward. (C) Moving both the upper and lower jaw forward.

Several different surgical procedures on the lower jaw are used to move the tongue forward. The procedures range from simply moving a small piece of bone forward at the tip of the jaw to moving the entire jaw by cutting through it on both sides and sliding it forward.

Other surgical procedures reposition the hyoid bone at the base of the tongue. A surgical team at Stanford University Medical Center that has pioneered this surgery performs a two-stage procedure involving UPPP, tongue advancement, and hyoid suspension, followed by upper/lower jaw advancement (40).

WHO CAN BE HELPED BY JAW SURGERY AND OTHER MAXILLOFACIAL SURGERIES?   It is not yet possible to predict precisely who will be helped by these surgeries. Many factors may influence the outcome, including not only the structure of the skull and soft tissue but also obesity, age, neuromuscular control of the airway, the presence of other sleep disorders, and, of course, the skill and experience of the surgical team.

Mandibular advancement is the simplest and safest of these procedures and is being used more often nationally, although its usefulness has not yet been fully established. It has been used in a relatively small number of patients with complicated apnea. An example is one patient who had a very small jaw and a small airway opening and for whom neither UPPP nor medication had helped. In this case, surgery did not completely eliminate his apnea, but reduced it by approximately half (41). As with many examples of sleep apnea surgery, whether the results are successful depends on if you define "success" as complete elimination of the apnea or if you are satisfied with elimination of half of the apnea and using CPAP to treat the apnea that remains.

Among 1,000 people with obstructive apnea studied at one sleep center, about 6 percent had an obviously malformed lower jaw and another 32 percent had a slightly short lower jaw (42). It is among these people that the best candidates for mandibular advancement surgery would probably be found, because their apnea is likely to arise in part from structural problems in the lower pharynx—a jaw and tongue positioned further back and lower than normal and an unusually small lower airway opening.

These complicated surgeries for sleep apnea should be planned as a team effort, involving the sleep specialist, an ENT specialist, the maxillofacial surgeon who will perform the actual mandibular surgery, and an orthodontist if teeth are to be repositioned (42).

The surgery itself is fairly safe if it is performed by an experienced surgeon. It is, however, performed under general anesthesia, which, as noted previously, is especially risky for people with breathing disorders.

WHAT ARE THE DRAWBACKS TO MAXILLOFACIAL SURGERY?   One major problem that may arise is difficulty with the healing of the jawbone because the blood supply to that area is not very generous. If the jaw is cut on both sides and moved forward (sliding osteotomy), the jaw may be wired closed during healing for about 6 weeks, which presents a significant inconvenience to the patient. In addition, orthodontics may also be required to reposition the teeth and realign the bite. The entire procedure is expensive and time consuming.

Another important drawback with this surgery should be considered. After mandibular surgery, the jawbone has a tendency to reposition itself backward again toward its original location. This happens over the course of several years in response to the powerful force of the tongue muscles, which are constantly pulling on the jawbone. Although some surgeons would disagree, other physicians have serious doubts about how long the results of this type of surgery can last.

Tracheostomy. Tracheostomy used to be a standard treatment for sleep apnea, but it has become much less common since the advent of CPAP. Today, it is performed primarily on two types of patients: people who are very sick from the effects of sleep apnea and who need immediate (sometimes emergency) treatment to save their lives, and those for whom other treatments have been unsuccessful. Tracheostomy has become the treatment of last resort; if all else fails, tracheostomy can be counted on to eliminate sleep apnea. In that sense, it is a very hopeful form of surgery. It also is fairly simple; however, it has some serious drawbacks.

WHAT IS A TRACHEOSTOMY? In a tracheostomy, a small opening is made into the trachea (windpipe) in the front of the neck just below the larynx (voice box). This opening may be permanent if tracheostomy is to be the permanent method of treating the person's sleep apnea. The opening can be surgically closed sometime in the future, if, for example, the patient switches to CPAP or some other therapy. The idea of a tracheostomy is to allow air to bypass the obstructions in the upper airway. The tracheostomy opening is closed with a plug during waking hours, and the person breathes normally through his nose and mouth. At night, however, the tracheostomy is left open, and breathing is done through the neck opening, unobstructed.

A tracheostomy tube usually is worn in the tracheostomy opening. This is a small, curved tube with a flange at the top. It is inserted through the tracheostomy opening and extends several inches down into the windpipe. The tracheostomy tube usually is worn permanently. The flange at the top helps hold the tube in place and protects the opening in the throat.

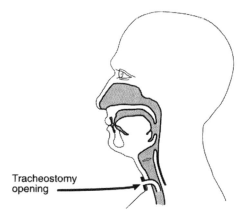

Tracheostomy opening

A tracheostomy with a tube in place. At night, the patient breathes through the tracheostomy opening, bypassing the obstruction in the patient's airway. During the day, the tube is closed with a plug, so that the patient can talk.

Tracheostomy surgery itself is not particularly risky, although it usually is done under general anesthesia, which may be risky.

Complications that may arise with tracheostomy fall into two categories. One involves the tracheostomy opening itself. In some cases, the opening tries to close itself up again. Other difficulties can result if the tissue around the opening heals incorrectly or becomes infected, damaged, or eroded. Several different surgical variations have been developed in an attempt to avoid such problems. Another complication of tracheostomy is respiratory infection, such as pneumonia. When a person breathes through a tracheostomy, air is inhaled virtually straight into the lungs, bypassing all the natural germ-filtering systems in the nose and upper airway. Consequently, bacteria, viruses, and other foreign objects can much more easily reach the lungs. Great care must be taken to prevent this from happening.

There may be a fair amount of pain, some swelling, and difficulty swallowing for several days after tracheostomy surgery. A tracheostomy tube is worn until the incision has healed. The tube is chosen for size and shape to fit the particular person and is not particularly uncomfortable to wear.

After a tracheotomy, the patient (at first with help from a family member) needs to follow a fairly rigorous, 24-hour postoperative program of taking care of the tracheostomy. This includes cleaning, suctioning, misting, and applying salt solution and antibiotics. Immediately after surgery, a suction machine must be used periodically to keep the tracheostomy tube clear of mucous secretions that could block the airway and prevent breathing. Mucus production decreases as time goes on, but a suction machine will be needed indefinitely for cleaning the tube and preventing mucus build-up. Cleanliness will always be extremely important to avoid introducing bacteria into the tracheostomy opening. The nurses and respiratory therapists should be explicit in teaching all these procedures to both patient and family.

WHO CAN BE HELPED BY A TRACHEOSTOMY?   Anyone with obstructive or mixed sleep apnea can be helped by a tracheostomy. Nowadays, the people chosen for tracheostomy usually have severe apnea with severe complications, including daytime drowsiness so severe that they are completely disabled (43). They may have tried other treatments and found them to be unsuccessful. They may have significant cardiac arrhythmias or other serious heart complications from severe sleep apnea. They may have extremely low oxygen levels in their blood.

Tracheostomy eliminates snoring, improves the quality of sleep, and virtually cures daytime drowsiness and apnea in nearly everyone who has the surgery. It greatly improves fatigue and morning headaches (43).

WHAT ARE THE DRAWBACKS TO TRACHEOSTOMY?   One of the main drawbacks of tracheostomy, and one reason it has fallen out of favor so quickly with the advent of CPAP, is the impact that it has on day-to-day lifestyle.

Most people need several weeks to months to learn to deal with the frustrations of tracheostomy hygiene and to adjust to their new image with a tracheostomy opening in the throat. A bout of depression commonly accompanies this adjustment period.

The severity and duration of the person's depression depend on the individual, on how well the person has been prepared for the appearance and the care of the tracheostomy, and on family support. The patient, spouse, and other close family members should be counseled about the surgical procedure, the care that is necessary afterward, and the likelihood of temporary depression. Talking with other people who have tracheostomies and are attending sleep apnea support groups, both before and after surgery, helps people to adjust more easily.

Most people who have had tracheostomies report that they do just fine once the initial adjustment period is over. They lead normal, active lives and generally do not seem to be bothered by their tracheostomies. However, they will always have to be careful about hygiene around the tracheostomy opening. And they must always take care that nothing enters the windpipe through the tracheostomy opening. For example, people with tracheostomies may not swim. Because the opening in the throat leads almost directly into the lungs, people with tracheostomies are in extreme danger from drowning and therefore must avoid not only swimming but also all water-related activities (water skiing, sailing, rafting, fishing from a boat) that might require swimming.

Other drawbacks involve the cosmetics of covering the tracheostomy opening. A small plate or shield is worn over the opening and is held in place by a cord around the neck. There is nothing inherently objectionable about its appearance, but many people choose to cover the tracheostomy plate with a turtleneck or a scarf.

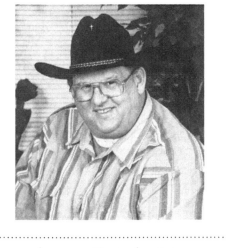

A person with a tracheostomy.

Another problem can be keeping the opening sealed during the day. Talking becomes difficult if there is air leakage. Coughing or sneezing can sometimes pop the seal and cause temporary embarrassment.

Other difficulties are problems that can arise from poor healing or erosion of the opening. To avoid such problems, it pays to find the most skillful surgeon you can (consider a plastic surgeon) and to follow carefully the postoperative instructions. Ask your doctor to answer any questions you may have and be persistent in asking for help in learning to deal with any follow-up problems.

Bariatric (Weight Loss) Surgery. Weight loss surgery has been called "behavioral surgery" (44) because it surgically enforces a change in a person's eating behavior that the person has been unable to accomplish by other means. The desired change in behavior is to reduce the amount of food the person consumes at any one sitting. This is done surgically by making the stomach smaller.

SURGICAL RISKS. Several types of bariatric surgery have been employed over the past 20 years. Bariatric surgery carries special risks because it is performed on obese people. The possibility of death from surgery is two to three times greater for obese people than for people of average weight (44). Consequently, it is important to weigh the risks carefully against the possible benefits that can reasonably be anticipated after surgery.

People who undergo gastric bypass usually are characterized as being morbidly obese. The average weight of 17 patients in one group was twice their recommended body weight (45). They were not having "cosmetic surgery" to lose weight; they were people whose lives are in danger because of their excessive weight and other complications.

The patients chosen for gastric bypass usually are screened to include only those who have already attempted to lose weight under carefully supervised weight-loss programs. The patient's psychological status often is evaluated as part of the screening process. Patients should understand the risks and behavioral changes that will be necessary for the bypass surgery to be successful.

Several versions of weight-loss surgery have been developed over the past 40 years. The most common surgical weight-loss procedures are gastric bypass and laparoscopic adjustable gastric banding.

GASTRIC BYPASS. This is the most common bariatric procedure performed today. In gastric bypass, the stomach is reduced in size, not by removing part of the stomach, but by placing a row of staples across it, dividing the stomach into a small upper pouch and a larger lower pouch. The upper pouch becomes the "new" stomach. It receives food from the esophagus and empties into a branch of the intestines that has been brought up and attached to it.

After surgery, food intake at any one time will always be restricted to approximately twice the volume of the "new" stomach, usually about 30 mL. This means that no more than about one-quarter of a cup of food can be eaten at a time.

Gastric bypass is major surgery (see illustration on page 97). It involves major organs (stomach and intestines) and some large arteries. It can be done either by opening the abdominal cavity or by laparoscopy (operating through small openings) (46). The risks of complications during surgery from either method are about equal. There are risks from anesthesia, other medications, surgical errors, and infection. During and after surgery the placement of a number of tubes will prolong the invasiveness of the procedure:

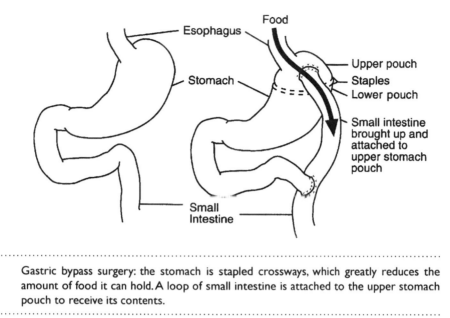

Gastric bypass surgery: the stomach is stapled crossways, which greatly reduces the amount of food it can hold. A loop of small intestine is attached to the upper stomach pouch to receive its contents.

a nasogastric tube for removing fluid from the stomach, catheters, intravenous hookups, and possibly an endotracheal tube for a ventilator.

Complications after bypass surgery can be significant. They may include infections, bowel obstruction, collapse of lungs, blood clots, and other after effects seen following abdominal surgery. The most common complication after gastric bypass is excessive vomiting (44).

Gastric bypass by open abdominal surgery typically requires a hospital stay of a week or more, considerable postoperative pain and discomfort, and an extended recovery period lasting from 4 to 5 weeks to months.

HOW EFFECTIVE IS GASTRIC BYPASS IN TREATING SLEEP APNEA? The average weight loss after gastric bypass is 65 percent to 70 percent of *excess* body weight (not total body weight), leveling off in 1 to 2 years (46). One study reported that most of their surgical patients' sleep apnea was significantly improved 6 months after surgery. Some patients had completely lost their symptoms. Many patients reported no daytime sleepiness or loud snoring. Changes in personality also were reported—greater responsiveness, fewer emotional problems, and less difficulty at work. A full year is needed for complete results, so during the 6 months following that report the patients in the study group might anticipate additional weight loss and further improvement in their apnea symptoms (45). In the long term, however, some people who have had gastric bypass surgery will return to their presurgery weight. The overall failure rate for gastric bypass surgery is reported to be from 30 percent to 50 percent (44).

Laparoscopic Adjustable Gastric Banding. "Lap-Band" surgery has been common in Europe and elsewhere but only was approved in the United States by the

Food and Drug Administration in 1991. This surgery, as its name suggests, is usually performed laparoscopically, so the surgery itself is not especially risky if it is done by an experienced surgeon. It involves placement of an inflatable band around the upper part of the stomach. Inflating the band restricts the stomach to a small pouch with a small drainage opening. A tube running from the band to a port outside the abdominal wall is used to adjust the inflation of the band, which has to be done several times per year.

HOW EFFECTIVE IS LAP-BAND SURGERY IN TREATING SLEEP APNEAS?   Statistics suggest that this surgery does not produce quite as great a weight loss as gastric bypass, achieving about a 50 percent loss of excess body weight (45). Among nine sleep apnea patients who had lap-band surgery, only three had their sleep apnea eliminated 18 months after surgery, but the remaining six did not improve at all (47).

Risks from lap-band surgery include those mentioned above for other bariatric surgeries plus potential damage to the esophagus or stomach, the possibility of infection from or malfunction of the inflatable band, and problems with the access port.

WHO CAN BE HELPED BY BARIATRIC SURGERY.   Bariatric surgery may be an effective and permanent—if radical—solution for severely obese apnea patients who are motivated to change their eating behavior, and whose physicians consider them to be good candidates for this type of surgery. The possible benefits should be carefully weighed against the significant potential risks.

Treatments for Central Apnea

Drugs

Drugs that stimulate the breathing reflexes are presently the most common treatments for central apnea. Unfortunately, most of the drugs have drawbacks that make them less than ideal. Some are not very effective; some work for a while, but the person may develop a tolerance to the drug; and some have undesirable side effects. Consequently, the drugs available today for treating central apnea should be considered temporary measures, and we must hope that research in this field will soon offer more acceptable alternatives.

Acetazolamide is the drug that has received the most attention. It makes the blood more acidic, which tends to stimulate the breathing reflex. Experiments have shown that acetazolamide can decrease the number of apnea events and result in a modest decrease in daytime sleepiness (48). Other studies are less enthusiastic (49), and there are reports of this drug leading to the development of obstructive apnea (50). More research is needed, but at the present time, acetazolamide is the most promising drug for the treatment of central apnea.

Another drug that has provided some improvement in central apnea is clomipramine, which is an antidepressant. It has been used on only a few patients and has resulted in improved sleep and respiration and fewer apnea events. However, some patients developed a tolerance to the drug after 6 to 12 months, after which it was no longer effective. In addition, clomipramine has some undesirable side effects, one of which is impotence (51).

A third drug that has been tried experimentally on central apnea is doxapram, which is a respiratory stimulant that normally is used only for the short term (1 or 2 hours at a time) to stimulate the breathing of patients who are recovering from anesthesia. It has never been recommended for long-term use, and it has some serious side effects, including hyperactivity, irregular heart rhythms, increased blood pressure, nausea and diarrhea, and urinary retention. It should not be used in people with heart disease, high blood pressure, or perhaps heart rhythm irregularities. These categories include many people who have serious complications from sleep apnea. It remains to be seen how useful this drug will be.

Other drugs that have been tried, with very little improvement in the central apnea, are aminophylline and theophylline, both of which are bronchodilators normally used to treat asthma and emphysema; almitrine, a breathing stimulant; naloxone, a drug that has been used to counteract the depression of the breathing reflexes that results from the use certain other drugs such as morphine and codeine; medroxyprogesterone, a hormone similar to the female hormone progesterone, which is known to stimulate respiration; and tryptophan, an amino acid that reportedly acts as an antidepressant. None of these medications has had dramatic effects on central apnea. All of them except tryptophan can have serious undesirable side effects (52,53).

Oxygen has also been tried with mixed results (54). It is useful in some severe cases in conjunction with CPAP and/or bi-level PAP (CPAP is described below).

With so many drugs in existence and new ones being developed each year, one hopes that drugs will soon be found that provide a specific treatment for people with central apnea without serious side effects. Much more vigorous research in this field is needed.

Breathing Devices

Newer Continuous Positive Airway Pressure (CPAP) Technology

Advances in technology have produced several variations on CPAP that can help people with central sleep apnea. A new generation of breathing devices, called auto-servo devices, can sample a person's breathing pattern and then mimic or improve upon the pattern when the person's breathing becomes abnormal.

People with central apnea, especially those who have tried CPAP without good results, should contact their sleep center and inquire about the new auto-servo–type CPAPs, currently available from both Respironics, Inc. (Pittsburgh, PA) and ResMed Corp. (San Diego, CA). In some cases, an auto-servo device can be used in place of a more cumbersome mechanical ventilator (see below).

For more information about CPAP and bilevel PAP, see the earlier section on treating obstructive sleep apnea.

The choice of treatment for central apnea should be made only after a thorough consultation with your sleep specialist.

Diaphragmatic Pacemaker

A diaphragmatic pacemaker works very much like a heart pacemaker. It uses tiny, rhythmic pulses of electric current to stimulate rhythmic muscle contractions. Diaphragmatic pacemakers were first developed to treat poliomyelitis patients whose breathing reflexes were damaged. However, the devices were never used much for this purpose because "iron lungs" were developed and the availability of the polio vaccine soon eliminated the need.

Since then some work has been done using diaphragmatic pacemakers in patients with spinal cord injuries whose breathing reflexes have been interrupted and in infants born with faulty breathing reflexes. A few diaphragmatic pacemakers have been tried on adult patients with central sleep apnea.

In theory, this seems like an ideal solution. Central apnea is essentially the absence of the nerve signal that goes to the diaphragm during sleep to tell it to breathe. A pacemaker used during sleep should be able to supply that signal. However, this technology has not advanced very rapidly, and the diaphragmatic pacemaker has not yet become widely available, probably partly because until recently the demand was not there. Demand may increase with better recognition of central sleep apnea.

Implanting the pacemaker requires delicate surgery to place a pair of tiny electrodes next to the phrenic nerves (the nerves that control the diaphragm). This is done either in the neck, using a local anesthetic, or in the chest cavity, under general anesthesia. Usually both nerves, one on each side of the body, are used rather than just one, which would only stimulate one side of the diaphragm. A small receiver also is placed underneath the skin during surgery (55,56). To use the pacemaker, a radio frequency generator is placed against the skin over the implanted receiver and radio frequency pulses stimulate the phrenic nerve.

Some problems and risks are involved in using a diaphragmatic pacemaker in a person with sleep apnea. One drawback is that it can cause obstructive apnea to emerge, which raises a new set of issues (57). The most serious risk is the possibility of damaging the phrenic nerve, either during surgery or at some later time. Of course, loss of both phrenic nerves would leave the person with a paralyzed diaphragm and unable to breathe well on his or her own. For this reason, the operation must be done with meticulous care to avoid the slightest damage to the nerves.

If you are considering this type of surgery, you would be wise to go to whatever lengths are necessary to locate a medical center that has an extensive history of installing and using diaphragmatic pacemakers and to find the surgeon who is most experienced with the procedure.

At present, a diaphragmatic pacemaker probably is not a practical treatment option for most people with central apnea, although it may be considered for some patients. As research is done and experience is gained, these devices may become a more attractive method of treatment.

Mechanical Ventilators

Several forms of mechanical breathing systems can be used to assist breathing during sleep by people with central apnea. These devices operate either by "positive pressure" (forcing air into the lungs in a rhythmic, breathing-like pattern) or by "negative pressure" (more or less mimicking the actions of the breathing muscles).

Positive-pressure ventilators operate by rhythmically pushing air into the airway through a tube. The air may be supplied through a face mask or nasal mask or through a tube that enters the body by way of a tracheostomy (an opening in the throat, described earlier in this chapter), or inserted through the nose or mouth.

A positive-pressure ventilator is less cumbersome than a negative-pressure ventilator, and its use is becoming more common as better ventilators and face masks become available.

A negative-pressure ventilator works differently. The best-known example of a negative-pressure ventilator probably is the "iron lung," which was developed in the 1930s to "breathe" for polio victims who had lost their breathing reflexes. Miniaturized versions of the iron lung have been developed that surround only the chest.

Mechanical ventilators have had their problems. The rhythm can be tricky to adjust; it must be regulated to breathe at the proper rate for the person using it. Blood oxygen and carbon dioxide levels must be carefully monitored to ensure safe and effective ventilator settings. A mechanical system that completely controls breathing is uncomfortable for people who are somewhat able to breathe on their own and need only occasional assistance.

The newest generation of ventilators are small and portable and minimize discomfort by allowing the person to breathe on his or her own as much as possible and to assist breathing only if the person stops breathing. These newer little ventilators can be effective for many people who have central apnea and are unable to sleep and breathe at the same time.

Mr. Kennedy, the patient we have been following, finally reached the decision point— what treatment would be best for him?

CASE STUDY

When he first heard about UPPP, Mr. Kennedy thought it had some appeal: a relatively simple operation that might eliminate his snoring, and maybe his sleep apnea, for good. However, his sleep specialist explained that he did not appear to be a very good candidate for UPPP.

Mr. Kennedy has a short jaw, so most of his obstructive sleep apnea probably arises from low in his throat. It probably would not be resolved by UPPP. In that light, the pain and risks of surgery didn't seem worthwhile.

With the advice of his sleep specialist, Mr. Kennedy decided on CPAP combined with weight loss.

Currently, Mr. Kennedy has been on CPAP for 22 years. He lost 20 pounds and is at his ideal weight. He exercises several times a week and feels better than he has ever felt in his life.

Mr. Kennedy travels a lot and takes his CPAP with him in a carry-on bag. Security people in airports often ask to look in the bag, but he has never been seriously hassled about it. He recently met an airport security guard who uses CPAP himself.

He has had occasional minor problems—colds, skin irritations, poorly fitting masks, equipment breakdown. But, like the pioneers that they are, Mr. Kennedy and other CPAP users learn to solve each problem as it arises. Meanwhile, CPAP machines have become more reliable and have shrunk to half the size and weight of the one he started with, and the masks have become smaller, lighter, and easier to wear.

Mr. Kennedy feels so much better now that he has never been seriously tempted to give up CPAP. He admits that he would rather not believe that he will have to use CPAP for the rest of his life. He was only 47 years old when he was diagnosed with sleep apnea, and he still thinks of himself as fairly young and vigorous. Sometimes he feels sorry for himself that he is saddled with this weird medical machine. But . . . CPAP does work.

He did briefly try an oral appliance, but an overnight monitor showed that he was still having apneas and a low blood oxygen level with the oral appliance in place. These results rule out an oral appliance and also suggest that maxillofacial surgery is unlikely to be effective. Under the circumstances, Mr. Kennedy is not willing to trade the simplicity and effectiveness of CPAP for the risks, discomforts, and unpredictable results of surgery. Maybe some better treatment for sleep apnea will come along someday. Meanwhile he will stick with CPAP.

◆ Summary

- The best treatment is the most conservative treatment that will succeed for you.
- Treatments for obstructive sleep apnea and mixed apnea:
  - Weight loss
  - Breathing devices such as CPAP
  - Oral devices such as tongue or jaw retainers
  - Medication
  - Surgery
- Before agreeing to surgery:
  - Ask a qualified sleep specialist to estimate the chances that surgery will eliminate your sleep apnea.
- Treatments for central apnea:
  - Medication
  - Breathing devices such as auto-servo devices, mechanical ventilators, and diaphragmatic pacemakers
  - Get a second opinion from an ENT surgeon who is experienced and skilled in the surgical treatment of sleep apnea.

Obesity and Sleep Apnea

- One of every three adults is obese.
- Obesity increases the odds of having obstructive sleep apnea.
- Sleep apnea contributes to the Metabolic Syndrome, a deadly combination of obesity, hypertension, high cholesterol, and diabetes.
- Treatment of sleep apnea and weight management are the keys to overcoming the Metabolic Syndrome.

Most people who are overweight have some degree of sleep apnea. However, you don't have to be obese to have sleep apnea, and some overweight people do not have sleep apnea. But the correlation between obesity and sleep apnea is very high.

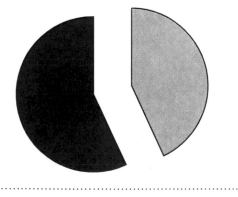

Fifty-seven percent of obese people have sleep apnea.

Obesity is important because it is a medical issue. It is not about clothing size or about losing weight. Obesity and sleep apnea together contribute to a host of medical disorders that lead to a downward spiral of worsening health.

Why Should You Care If You're Obese? The Sinking Spiral

The reasons obesity and sleep apnea tend to go hand in hand are threefold:

1. In obesity, fatty deposits accumulate within the layers of tissue in the neck. This causes constriction of the airway and contributes to snoring and sleep apnea.
2. In obese people, excess fatty tissue in the abdomen causes abnormal loading that interferes with the normal breathing mechanisms.
3. A sinking spiral develops. Sleep apnea destroys sleep and results in low oxygen during the nighttime and daytime drowsiness during the day. Repeated awakenings stress the sympathetic nervous system. This and the extra body weight contribute to hypertension. The body loses its ability to handle carbohydrates, slipping into insulin resistance, which equals adult-onset diabetes. Weight gain continues. Cholesterol levels increase and cardiovascular disease begins to take its toll. As sleep apnea worsens, excessive daytime sleepiness (EDS) also worsens. The person becomes less active, uses less energy, gains more weight, and further aggravates the apnea, diabetes, heart disease, becoming a candidate for, for example, heart attack and stroke.

The key is to break the cycle. Weight loss alone can do this, but it is extremely difficult to lose weight and keep it off in the face of all of the other challenges. Weight loss may be difficult or impossible to achieve as long as the sleep apnea is untreated. Treating the sleep apnea ends the spiral and opens the way to rebuilding total good health.

How Do You Know If You're Obese?

The simplest measure of central obesity is waist circumference. A waist larger than 40 inches in men or 34 inches in women is considered a sign of central obesity. Central obesity is a major cause of serious medical problems such as diabetes, sleep apnea, hypertension, high cholesterol, and heart disease. (Extra weight on hips or thighs is less of a medical concern.)

Another measurement is to compare your hip and waist sizes. If there is less than 4 inches between your hip size and your waist size, you have central obesity.

Body Mass Index (BMI) is a more precise measure of obesity (see illustration on page 105).

Body Mass Index is calculated by dividing body weight by the square of the height. You can find your precise BMI at the following National Institutes of Health web site, by typing in your height and weight: www.nhlbisupport.com/bmi/bmicalc.htm.

The Metabolic Syndrome and Sleep Apnea

The Metabolic Syndrome is a combination of disorders that often occur together and feed off of each other in a kind of downhill spiral of worsening health.

Body Mass Index Table

	Normal						Overweight					Obese										Extreme Obesity														
BMI	19	20	21	22	23	24	25	26	27	28	29	30	31	32	33	34	35	36	37	38	39	40	41	42	43	44	45	46	47	48	49	50	51	52	53	54
Height (inches)													Body Weight (pounds)																							
58	91	96	100	105	110	115	119	124	129	134	138	143	148	153	158	162	167	172	177	181	186	191	196	201	205	210	215	220	224	229	234	239	244	248	253	258
59	94	99	104	109	114	119	124	128	133	138	143	148	153	158	163	168	173	178	183	188	193	198	203	208	212	217	222	227	232	237	242	247	252	257	262	267
60	97	102	107	112	118	123	128	133	138	143	148	153	158	163	168	174	179	184	189	194	199	204	209	215	220	225	230	235	240	245	250	255	261	266	271	276
61	100	106	111	116	122	127	132	137	143	148	153	158	164	169	174	180	185	190	195	201	206	211	217	222	227	232	238	243	248	254	259	264	269	275	280	285
62	104	109	115	120	126	131	136	142	147	153	158	164	169	175	180	186	191	196	202	207	213	218	224	229	235	240	246	251	256	262	267	273	278	284	289	295
63	107	113	118	124	130	135	141	146	152	158	163	169	175	180	186	191	197	203	208	214	220	225	231	237	242	248	254	259	265	270	278	282	287	293	299	304
64	110	116	122	128	134	140	145	151	157	163	169	174	180	186	192	197	204	209	215	221	227	232	238	244	250	256	262	267	273	279	285	291	296	302	308	314
65	114	120	126	132	138	144	150	156	162	168	174	180	186	192	198	204	210	216	222	228	234	240	246	252	258	264	270	276	282	288	294	300	306	312	318	324
66	118	124	130	136	142	148	155	161	167	173	179	186	192	198	204	210	216	223	229	235	241	247	253	260	266	272	278	284	291	297	303	309	315	322	328	334
67	121	127	134	140	146	153	159	166	172	178	185	191	198	204	211	217	223	230	236	242	249	255	261	268	274	280	287	293	299	306	312	319	325	331	338	344
68	125	131	138	144	151	158	164	171	177	184	190	197	203	210	216	223	230	236	243	249	256	262	269	276	282	289	295	302	308	315	322	328	335	341	348	354
69	128	135	142	149	155	162	169	176	182	189	196	203	209	216	223	230	236	243	250	257	263	270	277	284	291	297	304	311	318	324	331	338	345	351	358	365
70	132	139	146	153	160	167	174	181	188	195	202	209	216	222	229	236	243	250	257	264	271	278	285	292	299	306	313	320	327	334	341	348	355	362	369	376
71	136	143	150	157	165	172	179	186	193	200	208	215	222	229	236	243	250	257	265	272	279	286	293	301	308	315	322	329	338	343	351	358	365	372	379	386
72	140	147	154	162	169	177	184	191	199	206	213	221	228	235	242	250	258	265	272	279	287	294	302	309	316	324	331	338	346	353	361	368	375	383	390	397
73	144	151	159	166	174	182	189	197	204	212	219	227	235	242	250	257	265	272	280	288	295	302	310	318	325	333	340	348	355	363	371	378	386	393	401	408
74	148	155	163	171	179	186	194	202	210	218	225	233	241	249	256	264	272	280	287	295	303	311	319	326	334	342	350	358	365	373	381	389	396	404	412	420
75	152	160	168	176	184	192	200	208	216	224	232	240	248	256	264	272	279	287	295	303	311	319	327	335	343	351	359	367	375	383	391	399	407	415	423	431
76	156	164	172	180	189	197	205	213	221	230	238	246	254	263	271	279	287	295	304	312	320	328	336	344	353	361	369	377	385	394	402	410	418	426	435	443

Source: Adapted from Clinical Guidelines on the Identification, Evaluation, and Treatment of Overweight and Obesity in Adults. The Evidence Report.

BMI Table. Find your height on the left side of the chart, read across to find your weight, and look at the top of that column to find your BMI.
National Institutes of Health, www.nhlbisupport.com/bmi/bmicalc.htm.

These disorders include:

- Adult-onset diabetes (also called type 2 diabetes), which includes:
  - Poor glucose tolerance (body does not process sugar properly)
  - Insulin resistance (body does not use insulin properly)
- Central obesity (extra weight is mostly on the belly, not on hips and thighs)
- High blood pressure (higher than 140/90 mm Hg)
- High cholesterol

A person who has three of these conditions has the Metabolic Syndrome.

Sleep apnea is also part of the Metabolic Syndrome picture. We know this because treatment of sleep apnea in a person with the Metabolic Syndrome can improve the person's insulin use (1), lower their blood pressure (2), and improve their cholesterol levels (3).

Untreated, the Metabolic Syndrome leads downhill, toward permanently damaged kidneys, heart, blood circulation, eyes, lungs, brain . . . and premature death (see illustration on page 106). This is why it is so important for obese people to find out whether they have sleep apnea, and get it treated.

CASE STUDY

Mrs. Baker had gained 50 pounds and felt increasingly exhausted. Her sleep was restless and unrefreshing, and her terrible, irregular snoring concerned her husband because she appeared to be gasping for air. Her doctor told her to lose weight and refused to refer her to a sleep center because "that's what they will tell you to do anyway."

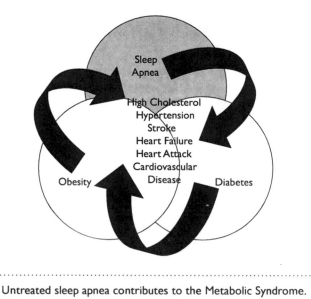

Untreated sleep apnea contributes to the Metabolic Syndrome.

Mrs. Baker joined a weigh- loss program and lost 50 pounds after spending $3,000. Her snoring improved a great deal, but it did not go away; and although her exhaustion had largely disappeared, she still felt drowsy when sitting, reading, or relaxing. Within 7 months her excess weight had returned, and with it her symptoms.

Another physician agreed to refer her to a sleep center. Moderately severe sleep apnea was diagnosed. Mrs. Baker was placed on CPAP, which eliminated her sleep apnea. On CPAP and with the help of a dietitian, she again lost the weight. Now at her ideal weight, she was again studied at the sleep center. To her dismay, she still had 50 percent of her sleep apnea unless she slept with CPAP.

Looking back, Mrs. Baker realized that after her initial and expensive weight loss, her apnea had continued to leave her fatigued and had decreased her activity level. As a result, her weight had increased; as she saw herself failing, she became depressed and ate more.

Now, using CPAP, Mrs. Baker is able to maintain her new weight.

CPAP eliminates the obstructive apnea, allowing more restful sleep, a better blood oxygen level, and improved metabolism which boost the person's energy level. The increase in energy and activity can then contribute to the weight loss effort.

The Obesity Hypoventilation Syndrome, or the "Pickwickian Syndrome"

The Pickwickian syndrome is a different combination of severe sleep apnea and obesity, in this case accompanied by a chronically decreased breathing pattern called *hypoventilation* and sometimes heart failure. This syndrome is found in approximately 5 percent of sleep apnea patients (4).

Mr. Roberts is a 45-year-old computer programmer and former college track star. He had always been active and energetic, with many outside interests.

Mr. Roberts first became aware that something was wrong with him in 1979. He realized that he felt tired a lot of the time. He had no energy. He became less and less active, and he started to gain weight. He began to take frequent naps. Eventually he began falling asleep at work. Fortunately, his boss liked and respected him, and he was sympathetic, although puzzled. He wondered if Mr. Roberts had a problem with alcohol or drugs and hoped that in time he would be able to work it out.

Between 1979 and 1985, Mr. Roberts changed from a trim, fun-loving, lively man into an overweight, lethargic, crabby near-invalid. He was asleep, or half asleep, nearly all the time. He also had developed heart problems. His doctor was stumped.

Mrs. Roberts was desperately worried. One day she heard by chance about a new sleep disorder center and talked her reluctant husband into making an appointment.

The sleep specialist immediately recognized Mr. Roberts's problem as a variety of sleep apnea. From the information in Chapter 1, you may recognize in Mr. Roberts one of the most common symptoms of sleep apnea—excessive daytime sleepiness.

Some clues from Mr. Roberts's past might have tipped you off further—his ability to fall asleep anywhere in any position and his loud snoring. When he was in the service, he was legendary; his snoring was so horrendous that his buddies often had to carry him outside in the middle of the night so that they could get some sleep. Many a morning Mr. Roberts woke up on his cot in the middle of the parade ground.

By the time he visited a sleep clinic, Mr. Roberts was showing all the symptoms of the Pickwickian syndrome.

In 1816, William Wadd, surgeon to King George III of England, connected obesity, lethargy, and breathing difficulty. He described three patients who were "suffocated by fat." In 1889, another medical man, A. Morison, reported a case of an obese, drowsy man whose drowsiness improved after he lost weight (5,6).

It was not until the 1950s that anyone came close to explaining what causes the Pickwickian syndrome. A respiratory physiologist was the first to suggest a cause-and-effect link between obesity and breathing difficulty. He proposed that obesity places an extra load on the respiratory system and suggested that this leads to lethargy and sleepiness (2), but he failed to connect sleep apnea with the total picture. Finally, in 1965, Gastaut demonstrated the relationship between sleep apnea and excessive daytime sleepiness.(7)

The term Pickwickian was first used as a medical term in an article by Bramwell in 1910. One of his patient's symptoms reminded him of the description and behavior of the fat boy, Joe, in Dickens's The Posthumous Papers of the Pickwick Club (1837). Joe was a "wonderfully fat boy" who was so sleepy he would fall asleep standing up.

To anyone who has no experience with the Pickwickian syndrome, this idea may seem far-fetched. But Charles Dickens was a keen observer of humankind and clearly depicted the most obvious symptoms:

- Marked obesity
- Daytime drowsiness
- Tendency to fall asleep during routine activities
- Snoring

Other features of the Pickwickian Syndrome that are less obvious to the casual observer are:

- Sleep apnea
- Bluish tone to face (cyanosis)
- Abnormal breathing reflexes
- Enlargement of right side of the heart
- Heart failure

What Causes the Pickwickian Syndrome?

The Pickwickian Syndrome is the result of several conditions coming together at once: sleep apnea, an abnormal breathing pattern, obesity, and usually some obstructive lung disease (4). Some people have a breathing reflex that is not very sensitive and allows the waste gas, carbon dioxide, to accumulate in their blood (see Chapter 6). This tendency becomes worse if the person's breathing is very shallow. Obesity causes shallow breathing by interfering with the work of the breathing muscles (7,8). This abnormally shallow breathing pattern becomes even worse when the person is lying down, and this in turn leads to such symptoms as frequent awakenings, sleep apnea, daytime sleepiness, low energy, and additional weight gain. A vicious circle develops, which is called the obesity-hypoventilation syndrome, or the Pickwickian Syndrome. The Pickwickian Syndrome may begin in childhood, and it can occur in adults who formerly were quite thin.

What Are the Effects of the Pickwickian Syndrome?

The Pickwickian Syndrome leads to the same problems that result from other kinds of sleep apnea. A person with Pickwickian Syndrome has fragmented sleep. Deep sleep and rapid eye movement (REM) sleep are reduced, sometimes nearly to zero. And because the person's shallow breathing does not take in sufficient oxygen during the night, a kind of slow asphyxiation occurs (7,9).

Excessive drowsiness during the daytime is common. People with Pickwickian Syndrome have a remarkable tendency to fall asleep whenever there is a moment's relaxation. They often fall asleep at their desks at work, in the middle of a conversation, or while driving a car.

Mr. Roberts tells of habitually driving to work and falling asleep in the parking lot. His coworkers would come out and find him, turn off the car, and guide him into his office, where he would spend the day sleeping at his desk. A Pickwickian doctor reported dozing off while examining a patient. He awoke to find his head resting on the patient's shoulder. A Pickwickian business executive finally sought treatment after falling asleep during a weekly poker game—he had drawn a full house (aces over kings) but then dropped off to sleep and missed the play (10).

Serious heart disease is closely associated with the Pickwickian Syndrome (7,9,10). In addition to the risks of hypertension, stroke, and coronary artery disease that accompany obesity, there are the risks of heart enlargement, arrhythmias, pulmonary complications, and heart failure that can result from sleep apnea. There is a relatively high rate of sudden death among the obese (9). The Pickwickian Syndrome should be treated seriously because in the long term it certainly is life threatening.

Treating the Pickwickian Syndrome

Continuous positive airway pressure (CPAP) combined with weight loss is the most conservative treatment. If CPAP is not able to eliminate the sleep apnea and low blood oxygen level, a temporary tracheostomy may be used (see Chapter 10).

The medical literature is mixed in its reports about the effectiveness of weight loss in reducing the symptoms of this syndrome. However, it may be that the more weight lost, the more likely it is that the person's apnea will improve. For any particular individual, there may be a critical weight above which the breathing difficulties of the Pickwickian Syndrome appear. Below that, weight improvement can be expected (10).

Mr. Roberts is a good example of a good outcome from the combination of CPAP and weighty loss.

CASE STUDY

Mr. Roberts was put on CPAP and a weight loss program. A year after beginning treatment for sleep apnea, Mr. Roberts was quite literally a different person. He had lost 100 pounds and was full of energy. He continued to steadily lose weight and was working at regaining his health. Thanks to a sympathetic boss, he still had his job. He was also remodeling his house (doing much of the work himself) and restoring several classic cars. He didn't hav e time to take naps.

Some people with Pickwickian Syndrome treated in this way appear to have a complete "remission." They can stop using CPAP, and they appear to be cured of sleep apnea (11).

Weight loss surgery (gastric bypass) is reported to be effective in treating the Pickwickian Syndrome, reducing sleep apnea to near zero and restoring deep sleep and REM sleep (9). However, gastric bypass surgery is not a trivial operation, and it should not be considered a conservative treatment option (see Chapter 10 for further information on treatment of sleep apnea).

◆ Summary

- Obesity is common among obstructive apnea patients.
    - The Meta[sws4]bolic syndrome is a combination of obesity, diabetes, hypertension, and treating the accompanying sleep apnea can help greatly.
- The Pickwickian Syndrome is a form of sleep apnea caused by a combination of obesity and a shallow, abnormally insensitive breathing mechanism.
- Symptoms of the Pickwickian Syndrome include:
    - Obesity
    - Daytime drowsiness
    - Falling asleep during routine activities
    - Snoring and sleep apnea
- Treatment includes CPAP and weight loss.

Sleep Apnea in Infants

- Infants are born with an immature breathing reflex, so infant breathing during sleep can vary a lot.
- Infants who struggle to breathe or stop breathing for longer than 20 seconds at a time may be at risk.
- Put infants to sleep on their back, and follow other guidelines to prevent sudden infant death syndrome (SIDS).
- A pediatric sleep specialist is best qualified to evaluate an infant's risk of sleep apnea or SIDS.

Breathing and Apnea in Infants

Normal, full-term infants are born with immature breathing reflexes. Variations in breathing during sleep are common—even normal—in infants. As explained by one authority, in infants "pauses in breathing are an integral part of normal respiratory behavior, are strongly influenced by age and sleep state, and do not of themselves constitute an abnormality" (1).

Pauses in breathing, known as apneas, during sleep are fairly common shortly after birth, and decrease with age as the breathing reflexes mature.

However, frequent or prolonged apneas are not normal and may be a sign of a breathing problem that should be brought to the attention of a doctor.

Premature infants' breathing reflexes are very immature, and these infants have even more apneas and longer apneas than full-term infants (2). Short apneas in premature infants are usually not considered to be a problem. However, apneas that are prolonged—for example, those that last more than 20 seconds in duration or are accompanied by decreases in heart rate and changes in color—are more concerning. It is often very difficult to predict which premature infants will have serious apneas during their first months at home. Some pediatric sleep and breathing specialists recommend that all premature infants with suspected apnea have a polysomnographic sleep study to help identify potential sleep/breathing problems (3).

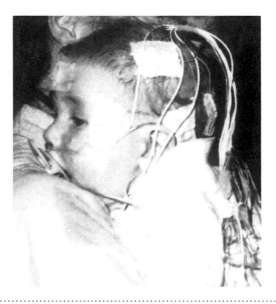

A child who is suspected of having a sleep disorder is prepared for a sleep test at a sleep center.

Experts disagree as to how much apnea should be considered a danger sign. Two or more apneas of more than 20 seconds during an 8-hour period would be considered prolonged apnea (1). Infants who show this kind of apnea during their first month of life should be considered at higher risk and need to be carefully watched.

Apparent Life-Threatening Events and Sudden Infant Death Syndrome

When an infant is found not breathing and blue, the situation is referred to as an apparent life-threatening event (ALTE). These infants may also be labeled near-miss sudden infant death syndrome (SIDS)."

Doctors sometimes can pinpoint the cause for an ALTE. Many conditions can cause breathing problems in infants, including congenital heart or lung abnormalities, structural abnormalities of the face or upper airway, bacterial or viral infections, abnormal metabolism, sedatives, seizures, and gastroesophageal reflux (regurgitation of the stomach contents) (4).

How does SIDS differ from ALTEs? They share characteristics, and there may be some overlap depending on your definitions. The peak in infant sleep apnea occurs 2 to 4 months after birth, which coincides exactly with the peak in SIDS (5).

One authority compared SIDS to a table littered with jigsaw puzzle pieces. "Our task is to fit [the pieces] together and to identify how many pieces are missing. One difficulty is that we don't know how many different jigsaw puzzles the pieces belong to" (6).

When an infant's apnea does not seem to be related to any of these causes, the diagnosis is simply "apnea of infancy."

A polygraphic sleep test can help diagnose the cause for unexplained apnea of infancy or ALTEs.

Risk Factors for SIDS

The following groups of infants are considered to have a higher risk of SIDS:

1. Infants who have experienced ALTEs
2. Infants experiencing long, observable apneas (lasting more than 20 seconds)
3. Premature infants who still have apneas when they are taken home from the hospital
4. Infants with a family history of SIDS
5. Infants sleeping on their stomach; soft bedding; fluffy objects in the crib
6. Smoking in the home (second-hand smoke)

Other factors include male sex and feeding practices. Male infants have a slightly higher chance of SIDS. Breast-feeding decreases the risk of SIDS (7).

However, the "high-risk" groups of infants account for only a small portion of SIDS victims (4,8). In the majority of SIDS cases, no previous risk factors were noted (8).

If you have an infant you think may fall into a higher risk category, you may want to talk to your pediatrician about your concern and ask for a consultation with a sleep specialist.

Preventing SIDS

1. The most important preventive measure is to always put a baby to sleep on its side or back, never on its stomach. "Back to Sleep" is the mantra. This is contrary to Grandma's long-standing practice of putting an infant to bed on its stomach. Nevertheless, data show that on-the-back sleeping significantly decreases the risk of SIDS. Since 1992, when the American Academy of Pediatrics made this recommendation, there has been a 38 percent decrease in the incidence of SIDS (9). Although this is not absolute proof of the cause of SIDS, it does suggest a strong relationship between the on-the-stomach (supine) sleep position and SIDS.
2. Parents should remove fluffy toys and loose bedding (for example, sheepskin) from the crib. A baby can suffocate if its face becomes buried in these objects.
3. Second-hand smoke from adults smoking in the home is also strongly correlated with SIDS. Make your baby's home a smoke-free environment.
4. Every adult who cares for your infant should know cardiopulmonary resuscitation (CPR).

5. Talk with a pediatric sleep specialist if you think your baby may be at risk for SIDS.

Apnea Monitors: Coping with Risk

A number of electronic apnea monitors are available for use at home in selected situations. However, they are not foolproof.

Apnea monitors are sensors that are either placed under the baby's mattress or attached to the baby's abdomen. If breathing stops for a selected period of time, usually 20 seconds, the monitor signals the parents by ringing a bell and flashing a light. However, the monitors can be fooled into giving false alarms, often as 25 percent to 50 percent of the time. A lot of false alarms can be discouraging for the parents and may tempt them to turn off the monitor (10).

The fact that monitors can also give a false-negative response is more serious: failing to indicate that breathing has stopped when it has. This can happen if the baby stops breathing, but the heartbeat, which becomes stronger when breathing stops, is still felt by the monitor. Additionally, muscle movements during an obstructive apnea can be misinterpreted as breathing. In either case, the alarm might not go off until all motion has stopped, by which time brain damage or death may have occurred (10).

Despite these drawbacks, there are cases in which a monitor might be helpful: for a premature infant who seems susceptible to prolonged apnea, for an ALTE or "near-miss" infant whose pediatrician has ruled out other known causes of infant apnea; and for some siblings of SIDS victims who are considered to be at high risk and whose parents need reassurance (10).

The monitor should be used for as long as the physician and parents think it is necessary. This may be from 3 to 5 months and until the child reaches an age the physician regards as safely beyond the risk of SIDS. Or the physician may wait until the child passes through an adequate alarm-free period and appears able to tolerate immunizations and respiratory infections without breathing difficulty (4).

If an apnea monitor is to be used, the baby should be examined by a physician who is familiar with these devices in order to decide on the best type of monitor to use. In addition, a 24-hour support service should be arranged through the doctor or the hospital in case of equipment breakdown.

Finally, it is extremely important that everyone who cares for the infant (parents, grandparents, other relatives, babysitters) be trained in CPR. If you have not had CPR training, ask your doctor to arrange it for you or ask your local Red Cross for a schedule of their classes.

Treating Infant Sleep Apnea

Most infant apnea disappears as the infant matures. SIDS is uncommon after age 6 months. If apnea continues beyond 6 months, various treatment options, including nasal CPAP, may be suggested by a sleep specialist (see illustration on page 115) (11,12).

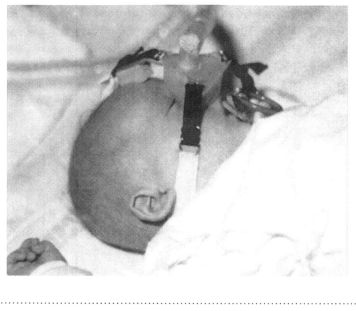

A 6-week-old infant being treated with CPAP.

A pediatrician specially trained in pediatric sleep disorders is best qualified to evaluate infant sleep problems. Sleep studies performed on infants need to be set up and evaluated according to different criteria than are used in adult sleep apnea. Furthermore, if CPAP therapy is recommended, the pediatric sleep specialist and staff will be able to work with the family and the pediatrician to make sure the therapy works effectively.

Long-Term Risks of Sleep Apnea

Treating infant sleep apnea is important not only to protect the infant but also in the long term. Untreated infant sleep apnea can affect the infant's growth, developing brain, and heart (13). Therefore, it is doubly important to discuss your concerns about childhood sleep-disordered breathing with a sleep specialist.

◆ Summary

- To help prevent SIDS: put an infant to sleep on its back; remove fluffy bedding and toys from the crib; do not allow smoking in the home.
- Sleep apnea can result in infant death but may be the cause of many cases of SIDS.
- Infants who are premature and still have apneas at the time they are sent home from the hospital, who have had an ALTE or have been diagnosed as having "apnea of infancy," or who are younger siblings of SIDS infants are considered to have a higher risk of SIDS.

- Infants who stop breathing during sleep or whose breathing during sleep is noisy should receive a thorough evaluation, including a sleep study.
- An apnea monitor may be indicated for high-risk infants.
- Treatment of sleep apnea depends on the cause of the sleep apnea.
- Treatment of sleep apnea will prevent problems with growth and development.
- Consult a pediatric sleep specialist if you suspect sleep apnea in an infant.

Snoring and Sleep Apnea in Older Children and Adolescents

- Snoring in children is not normal.
  - Snoring associated with sleep apnea can retard development, learning, and memory
  - Find and eliminate the cause of snoring, the sooner the better.
- Sleep apnea in older children usually is caused by:
  - Enlarged tonsils and adenoids
  - Obesity
- A tonsillectomy/adenoidectomy may eliminate sleep apnea in about four of five children, but the remaining one-fifth may need further treatment.
- CPAP therapy success demands expert care by a pediatric sleep medicine team.
- To locate a pediatric sleep medicine specialist, contact the American Academy of Sleep Medicine, www.aasmnet.org.

Childhood Snoring Is Not Normal

Snoring in children is not normal. Pediatricians may tell parents not to worry about snoring because the child will outgrow it. Parents should not wait for this to happen because snoring can slow down the normal course of growth and development.

In fact, children are much more vulnerable to the damaging medical consequences from snoring and even mild obstructive sleep apnea (OSA) than are adults. Obstructive sleep apnea can affect a child's heart and developing brain. Snoring and sleep apnea can cause memory, learning, and behavior problems that resemble attention deficit hyperactivity disorder (ADHD): hyperactivity, irritability, difficulty paying attention, and acting out in school (1–4).

One researcher compared the school performance of two groups of children who snored or had sleep apnea and were underachieving. The group of children who were treated with an adenotonsillectomy had a marked improvement in their school performance compared with the group who were not treated (5).

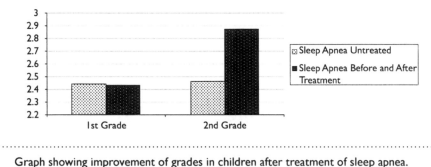

Graph showing improvement of grades in children after treatment of sleep apnea.

The American Academy of Pediatrics recommends that all children be screened for snoring (6). If a child snores loudly and often, the cause of the snoring should be identified and eliminated, before the snoring has a chance to affect learning or development.

Childhood Sleep Apnea Has Become More Common

Sleep apnea in older children is more common today than it was a generation ago for two reasons:

1. Tonsillectomies and adenoidectomies are much less common now, so many more children today have enlarged tonsils and adenoids.
2. Obesity is much more common now. One of every four or five children is obese, and obesity is associated with snoring and sleep apnea.

It is important to identify childhood sleep apnea early, and to treat it as soon as possible. Sleep apnea can negatively affect learning, behavior, mood, metabolism, and development, as well as the immune and cardiovascular systems.

Enlarged tonsils and/or adenoids are the most common causes of sleep apnea in children. However, tonsillectomy and adenoidectomy are not effective in curing 30 percent of children (7).

CASE STUDY

Jody was a 10-year-old girl who had been snoring terribly for 3 years. She also made snorting noises in her sleep. She was tired and short-tempered during the day, both at home and at school. Her tonsils were large, but her pediatrician did not believe in taking out tonsils unless they were regularly becoming infected. He told the family she would outgrow this.

The family physician suggested an evaluation at a sleep center. The sleep test revealed that Jody had severe apnea, with 40 apneic events per hour. She had a tonsillectomy and adenoidectomy, her symptoms disappeared, and her temper and school grades improved markedly.

Causes of Sleep Apnea in Children

The causes of sleep apnea in children are similar to those in adults:

- Obstructive sleep apnea occurs as a result of either a narrow or blocked airway. Airway blockage can occur as a result of nasal obstruction from a deviated septum or from allergies, large tonsils or adenoids, large soft palate, small lower jaw, and other structural features of the mouth, jaw, or throat that result in a narrow upper airway. Obesity also is a contributing factor.
- Central apnea results from an abnormal breathing drive in the brain.
- Mixed apnea is a combination of central and obstructive apnea.

Symptoms of Sleep Apnea in Children

Snoring is the most obvious symptom of childhood sleep apnea. Heavy snoring, accompanied by loud gasping and snorting, alternating with silence, is a sign of obstructive apnea.

Restless sleep, mouth breathing, and unusual sleep positions are other possible signs of sleep apnea. A child who is having trouble breathing often will thrash about, sit up, or sleep with the head held backwards and the neck stretched out in a position that helps to keep the airway open.

The behavioral symptoms of sleep apnea in children often are quite different from those seen in adults. Do not assume that a child with a sleep disorder must appear sleepy!

Sleepy children may actually become "wound-up," hyperactive, or aggressive. In fact, children have been diagnosed with attention-deficit hyperactivity disorder (ADHD) when their primary problem was sleep apnea or another sleep disorder. Improved behavior on stimulant medicines like methylphenidate (Ritalin) does not prove that the child has ADHD, since a child with a sleep disorder will also behave better on Ritalin. Furthermore, many children with ADHD also have sleep disorders, the treatment of which may result in improved behavior. A child who is hyperactive and who snores or has restless sleep should be evaluated by a sleep specialist to determine whether he has sleep apnea or another sleep disorder that needs to be treated.

Some children with sleep apnea may simply appear quiet, withdrawn, or pathologically shy. Their "good" behavior may not be perceived as a sign of a problem, even by their family.

Children whose apnea arises primarily from obesity are most likely to have the signs you would expect in an adult—daytime sleepiness and lethargy (7).

As with snoring, poor performance at school—poor concentration, underachievement, behavioral problems—is one of the most typical signs of sleep apnea. It is estimated that two-thirds of the children who are eventually diagnosed as having sleep apnea are not identified until their parents are alerted to a problem by school authorities.

Other possible signs of sleep apnea are bed-wetting, morning headache, and cardiovascular problems, such as high blood pressure and arrhythmias (heartbeat abnormalities) (8,9).

Untreated sleep apnea in children is likely to become worse and in time leads to the same kinds of cardiovascular and respiratory complications that are seen in adults. It should be considered life threatening in the long term. Furthermore, it is impossible to overstate the disadvantages these children may suffer as a result of poor performance in school. The consequences of inattention, poor concentration, poor memory, and behavioral problems can affect a child for the rest of his or her life, so no time should be lost in treating sleep apnea.

If your pediatrician or family physician is not familiar with sleep apnea, he may fail to recognize its signs. You might want to make a tape recording of the sounds of your child's snoring and ask your doctor to refer you to a sleep specialist. It is important that a child who is suspected of having sleep apnea be thoroughly tested by a sleep specialist and that treatment be started as soon as possible.

Testing for Sleep Apnea in Children

When Should a Child See a Sleep Specialist?

An appointment with a pediatric sleep specialist is in order:

- If a doctor suggests a sleep medication for the child (The FDA has not approved most sleeping pills for use by children.)
- If sleep apnea is suspected
- If bedtime behavior is very disruptive
- If the child has a medical or psychological problem that makes sleep difficult

Evaluation of a child for sleep apnea and other sleep disorders (see Chapter 12) should be done at an accredited sleep center, preferably by a board certified pediatric sleep specialist. Children are more difficult to diagnose and can easily be misdiagnosed by doctors who are inexperienced at performing pediatric sleep studies, or by sleep laboratories that do not have the appropriate laboratory technology. The following cases show that inadequate testing can easily lead to misdiagnosis and inappropriate treatment.

CASE STUDY

Billy was 10 years old, and his teacher reported that he was having trouble paying attention in school. He was crabby and was a restless sleeper. No medical problems were identified other than allergies, which caused nasal breathing and enlarged tonsils. Billy's parents insisted on testing for a sleep disorder, and a limited test for breathing during sleep was done in their home. The results were negative and "proved" that there was no sleep problem. Unconvinced, the parents took Billy to an accredited pediatric sleep specialist, where a comprehensive sleep study showed mild sleep apnea and that had been missed with the simple home test.

CASE STUDY

Becky was 8 years old and had been waking up yelling and rhythmically shaking her legs. She was tired and appeared confused the next day. This happened a few times a month and was very disturbing to her parents. They took her to a neurologist, but nothing was found. She then was studied at a sleep center where the specialist recognized that she had a seizure disorder. Her parents agreed to start her on medications, and her episodes stopped entirely.

CASE STUDY

Mary was 7 years old and had been waking up moaning, with her legs rigid and shaking. She appeared confused, and her parents thought she looked as if she were having seizures. Her neurological evaluation was negative, but she had some "abnormalities" in her electroencephalogram (EEG). She was diagnosed as having seizures and was given medications. She developed a severe rash. Her parents eventually took her to a pediatric sleep specialist who diagnosed a night terror disorder that mimicked seizures. The seizure medication was stopped, and her spells gradually disappeared.

Diagnostic testing for sleep apnea in children should include a thorough physical examination, with special emphasis on the anatomy of the face, neck, and upper airway. This may include a fiberoptic examination of the airway.

An x-ray–type image of the child's head may also be needed. Computerized tomography (CT scan, especially fast CT) and magnetic resonance imaging (MRI) are other options, but both of these procedures are more expensive. Consult your doctor about which of these options is most appropriate.

An overnight sleep test should be performed to confirm the presence of sleep apnea, to measure the severity of the disorder, and to rule out other disorders. A multiple sleep latency test (MSLT) also may be done to measure the degree of sleepiness.

Pediatric Sleep Studies Use Pediatric Standards

The results of a child's sleep study should be evaluated a little differently from those of an adult. The standards for evaluating childhood sleep apnea have been evolving as more is learned about the disorder in children. The number of apneas and hypopneas (partly obstructed breaths) per hour of sleep, known as the Apnea-Hypopnea Index (AHI), is less than 1.5/hour in normal children. In contrast, an AHI that is greater than

5 per hour of sleep is considered a sign of mild sleep apnea in adults, but in children it might be considered more serious (10).

This is why it is wise to look for a sleep specialist who is experienced with pediatric sleep disorders.

Treating Obstructive Sleep Apnea in Children

Surgery

Because most obstructive apnea in children is due to enlarged tonsils and adenoids, the most frequent treatment is simply to remove them. The operation has some risk but is fairly routine. However, about one of five children who have a tonsillectomy and adenoidectomy will have persistent sleep apnea and need further treatment.

Some children with severe sleep apnea may be candidates for uvulopalatopharyngoplasty (UPPP) or mandibular surgery (described in Chapter 10).

However, many of the surgeries performed on adults are not appropriate in a child.

CPAP

Continuous positive airway pressure (CPAP) is the treatment of choice for children whose obstructive sleep apnea cannot be resolved by a tonsillectomy and adenoidectomy. Children with an abnormally small jaw structure may be placed on CPAP until they are old enough (teenaged) for surgery to be effective.

CPAP in children is most successful when the therapy and follow-up are carried out by pediatric sleep medicine staff who are well trained in the "art" of CPAP therapy in children. Family and child should all be educated about the importance of the therapy, and if the child is old enough, she should understand how the mask and equipment works.

It is impossible to overemphasize the importance of the trained pediatric sleep medicine staff in achieving successful CPAP use in children (11,12). If you feel you or your child is not receiving adequate attention, do not hesitate to insist on better care, or find a sleep center that has more experience with pediatric care.

Children of any age can successfully use CPAP, provided the parents and children are well informed, cooperative, and have access to skillful follow-up staff.

Weight Management

Weight loss is difficult but usually is helpful if obesity is contributing to the cause of sleep apnea. Weight loss works best if the whole family is involved in a program of weight management and counseling (7). However, because of the time required for significant weight loss and the difficulty of maintaining the lower weight, an overweight child with sleep apnea probably should have concurrent therapy with CPAP until weight management is well underway.

Regardless of treatment, a follow-up sleep study is important to confirm that the therapy has been effective at eliminating the sleep apnea.

Good Sleep Habits Also Help

Establishing good sleep habits will help any child (and parents) to enjoy the benefits of better sleep, not only during childhood but throughout life. Parents should be in charge of a child's sleep routine, and would do well to enforce the following bedtime routine.

- Sufficient sleep duration, appropriate to the child's age:
  - Preschool: 11 hours per night
  - Ages 7–11:   10 hours per night
  - Adolescents: 9 hours or a little more every night (not just weekends)
- A regular bedtime appropriate to the child's age, and a regular wake-up time.
- A calming, 20- to 30-minute bedtime routine ending up in bed
- A light bedtime snack if the child enjoys one
- No caffeine (colas, coffee, tea) within 4 hours of bedtime
- No getting "wound-up" with energetic activities within an hour of bedtime (including TV, video games, exercise)
- No electronic media in the bedroom (TV, computer, phone, video games)
- Some outdoor exercise every day (sunlight, especially in the morning, helps to regulate the sleep-wake cycle)

◆ Summary

- Sleep apnea in older children usually results either from enlarged tonsils or adenoids or from obesity.
- Consult a sleep specialist if you suspect sleep apnea in a child. The diagnosis can be tricky because the symptoms of sleep apnea in children may not appear to be related to sleep.
- Treatment depends on the cause of the sleep apnea, as discussed in this chapter.
- Tonsillectomy and adenoidectomy can be effective, but 30 percent of children will still have apnea and need further treatment. Insist on a postsurgical assessment of your child's breathing.
- Long-term follow-up should include periodic parental observation to be sure symptoms do not return.

Women and Sleep Apnea

- Before menopause, sleep apnea in women is only one-third as common as in men.
- After menopause, a woman's chance of having sleep apnea triples.
- The signs of sleep apnea in women are:
    - Snoring (28 person of women snore)
    - Waking up coughing or choking
    - Stopping breathing during sleep
    - Feeling fatigued or sleepy during the day
    - Weight gain
- Check the BMI table (see illustration on page 105) to see whether you are obese.
- If your doctor does not suggest a sleep study, and you suspect sleep apnea, you should schedule one yourself.

Women's sleep has been studied only since the 1990s, so there is still much to learn. But it is already clear that women's sleep is more complicated than men's because of the physiological changes that occur with the onset of puberty and continue across the woman's lifespan: the menstrual cycle, pregnancy, childbirth, menopause, and beyond.

Women Have More Sleep Problems than Men

Women have the capacity to be easily awakened, but also experience more deep sleep than men. Consequently, on the whole, women's sleep may be more restorative than men's sleep. One theory proposes that evolution may have favored a woman's ability to alternate between awakening easily in order to care for an infant, and then grabbing a short, deep, "power sleep" before being awakened again for infant care (1).

Women have more problems than men with insomnia and fatigue. Insomnia is three to four times more common among women. The hormone fluctuations of the menstrual cycle are responsible for variations in a woman's ability to fall asleep and stay asleep. Fragmented sleep and insomnia are characteristic of the premenstrual phase, while in the postmenstrual phase, falling asleep usually is easier. Women after menopause and older men both may experience lighter sleep, and may sleep fewer hours. This is discussed in the next chapter.

During the hormonal fluctuations of the menopause years, a woman's sleep may be fragmented many times during the night by hot flashes. Most hot flashes awaken the woman, and the result is daytime fatigue and potentially some negative effects on overall health (2).

Pregnancy plays havoc with sleep, and following childbirth a woman will never again experience as high a quality of sleep as she knew before pregnancy.

Restless legs syndrome (RLS) and periodic limb movement in sleep (PLMS) are also more common in women, and especially likely to appear during pregnancy.

Sleep Apnea Looks Different in Women

For years, sleep apnea was considered a "men's disorder." The prevalence in men appeared to be 10 times that of women. But then someone looked more closely at the numbers and found that the ratio was closer to three to one, men to women. Twenty-eight percent of middle-aged women snore habitually compared with 44 percent of men. After menopause, the rate of sleep apnea triples (3). Sleep apnea no longer belongs just to the men!

One reason sleep apnea has been underrecognized in women is because women may not have the same symptoms as men. Men tend to snore loudly and have apneas off and on throughout the night. Women also snore (one of every four women snores), but it tends to be limited mostly to rapid eye movement (REM) sleep.

Also, women may exhibit a quiet variation of sleep apnea called upper airway resistance syndrome (UARS). UARS is more subtle than snoring, but its long-term effects are equivalent to those of obstructive sleep apnea, because in UARS there is a struggle to breathe, a disruption of sleep, and low oxygen levels in the blood as seen in obstructive sleep apnea. Like obstructive sleep apnea, UARS is treated with continuous positive airway pressure (CPAP).

UARS and sleep apnea can cause hypertension and contribute to the development of diabetes.

Women, Obesity, and Sleep Apnea

One-third of adults are obese, and overweight women are more likely to have sleep apnea along with the other risks that accompany excess weight. Obesity plus high blood pressure, diabetes, and high cholesterol add up to the metabolic syndrome, a deadly combination of diseases with a high mortality rate that should be treated from every angle possible. Metabolic syndrome is discussed in Chapter 11.

Obstructive sleep apnea contributes to the metabolic syndrome, and treatment of the sleep apnea should be part of a treatment package aimed at weight management, controlling diabetes, and managing blood pressure and cholesterol levels.

How do you know if you're obese? The standard Body Mass Index (BMI) table (see illustration on page 105) considers anyone with a BMI higher than 25 to be obese. If your waist is less than 4 inches smaller than hips, it is a sign of "central" obesity, a higher cardiovascular risk than the hips-and-thighs pattern of excess weight.

If you or a loved one fall into these categories, you would be wise to find out if you have sleep apnea and to ask your doctor for referral to wellness programs that specialize in managing weight and lowering cardiovascular risks. Most medical centers offer such programs, and insurance often will pay for it.

Sleep Apnea Can Cause Complications During Pregnancy

Pregnancy frequently brings women their first experience with sleep apnea. As many as one-quarter of pregnant women have episodes of sleep apnea, particularly during the third trimester of pregnancy.

A little light snoring probably is not a problem. However, heavy snoring is linked with a higher risk of complications in pregnancy (4). In particular, snoring can increase the chances of hypertension and preeclampsia (4,5).

Heavy snoring by the mother can also retard the growth of the fetus (4).

Consequently, if a woman is snoring heavily during pregnancy, or if breathing stops during sleep, a visit to a sleep specialist is definitely in order. CPAP therapy can be prescribed for use during pregnancy, and stopped if it is no longer needed after the birth of the baby.

Sleep Apnea Is More Common After Menopause

If hot flashes are not disturbing enough, menopausal women may have sleep apnea to look forward to. The chances of having sleep apnea triple after menopause. Otherwise normal women of average body weight who have never had a prior sign of sleep apnea can find themselves waking up during the night with such symptoms as coughing or choking, feeling fatigued during the day, gaining weight, and becoming depressed.

During and after menopause, half of women have complaints about their sleep. In the past, these sleep problems would have been considered "just a normal part of life" after menopause. Hormone replacement therapy has been prescribed under the assumption that low or fluctuating hormones are causing sleep problems. Now we know that hormone replacement does not lessen hot flashes or other sleep problems (6).

Symptoms of disturbed sleep after menopause should be taken seriously, as potential signs of sleep apnea or another treatable sleep disorder. When in doubt, a sleep study will provide the answer. One researcher on women's sleep warns other physicians (7):

> Signs and symptoms that would normally trigger a full sleep evaluation in premenopausal women should be taken as seriously in menopausal women.

In other words, do not wait for your family doctor to suggest a sleep study. The idea may never occur to them.

◆ Summary

- Women are more likely than men to have insomnia, but about one-third as likely to have sleep apnea.
- Sleep apnea increases after menopause.
- Obesity or weight gain increases the likelihood and severity of sleep apnea.
- Sleep apnea often accompanies the metabolic syndrome (obesity, diabetes, hypertension, and high cholesterol), which should be treated with a combination of CPAP and management of weight, diabetes, cholesterol, and blood pressure.
- If you awaken coughing or choking during the night, or stop breathing during sleep, you may have developed sleep apnea and should arrange to have a sleep study.

Sleep Apnea and Seniors

- Older people's sleep normally is lighter and more fragmented.
- Sources of sleep disturbance include sleep apnea, movement disorders, pain, respiratory problems, and depression.
- If you have signs of sleep apnea, schedule a sleep study.
- Good sleep habits can improve the quality of sleep.
- Exposure to morning light (outdoors, or indoors with a light box) regulates the sleep-wake cycle, and can help seniors to sleep through the night and avoid early awakening.

Sleep in Older People

We often assume that it is normal for older people to get less sleep during the night than younger people. This assumption often is further explained by the assumption that "older people don't need as much sleep." In fact, both of these assumptions are open to question.

It is true that people over 50 years of age typically do get less than 7 hours of sleep during the night compared with 8 hours for people 19 to 30 years old. This is partly because older people awaken more often during the night and partly because they usually wake up earlier in the morning (1). However, older people also appear to take more frequent daytime naps than young people, so an older person's total amount of sleep during a 24-hour period may be very close to the 8 hours obtained by a younger person (2).

However, the quality of sleep that older people get is not as good as it is in younger people. From reading Chapter 6, you know that the quality of the sleep is diminished when a night's sleep is broken up by wakefulness. Older people's sleep is lighter and more fragmented by periods of wakefulness than is the sleep of younger people.

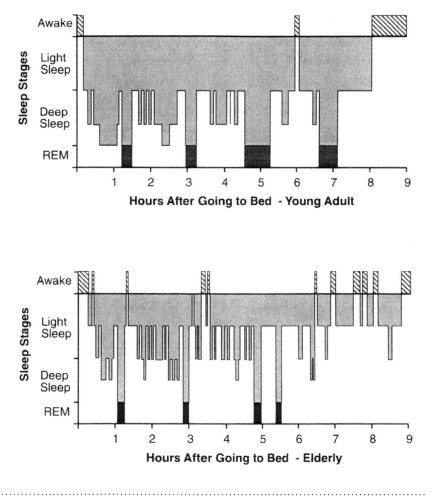

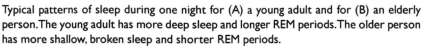

Typical patterns of sleep during one night for (A) a young adult and for (B) an elderly person. The young adult has more deep sleep and longer REM periods. The older person has more shallow, broken sleep and shorter REM periods.

Older people experience less deep sleep (see illustration on page 130). They get almost as much REM sleep as younger people, but it is less intense (1).

Older people may be attempting to compensate for sleep lost during the night by napping. In some individuals, naps may make up for the amount of sleep lost, but they do not make up for the loss of sleep quality at night. In fact, in some people, naps may simply compound the problem, both by making the person less sleepy at night and by confusing the person's internal clock.

Older people spend
 • more time awake in bed or in light sleep
 • less time in deep sleep

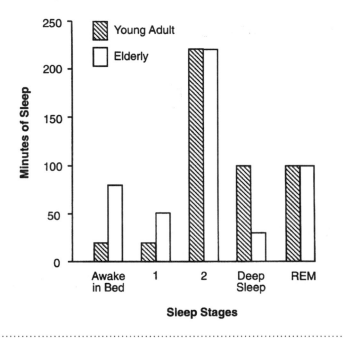

Comparison of the amount of time young people and older people spend in each stage of sleep.

The significance of these differences between the sleep of older people and younger people is not understood. No one knows exactly why we need deep sleep and REM sleep, so the meaning of the decrease in these stages of sleep with age remains to be discovered.

Myths about Sleep and Aging

The majority of older people are healthy and have few, if any, complaints about sleep disturbances. Even though their sleep may be more fragmented than it was when they were younger, they do not appear to be unduly bothered by it. However, some older people do have serious sleep problems. Unfortunately, they may be discouraged from seeking help by certain myths about sleep and aging.

 • Feeling sleepy is not "just part of getting old," Do not rationalize that being sleepy during the day is "just part of being old" and do not accept this explanation from a family physician either. If you are drowsy to the point that it affects your ability to drive alertly for at least an hour, to read for 30 minutes or more, or to sit and socialize with family, the odds are that you may have a treatable sleep disorder.

- Disturbed or poor sleep is not normal. Do not accept explanations that claim that disturbed or poor nighttime sleep is "normal." Although most elderly people agree that their sleep is not what it used to be, most do not believe that poor sleep is significantly interfering with how they feel or function.

If you think your quality of life is being diminished by sleeping difficulties, do not hesitate to seek help and do not be discouraged by those who would make light of your complaints.

Reasons for Disturbed Sleep in Older People

Sleep Apnea

Sleep apnea is one of several medical conditions that can seriously interfere with the sleep of older people. Sleep apnea has been reported in as many as 30 percent of the healthy elderly adults who have been studied (2,3). It probably results from the gradual loss of tone in the muscles in the upper airway that occurs with increasing age.

The sleep apnea seen in healthy older people is usually very mild or moderate. In many cases, it is not severe enough, or is barely severe enough, to qualify as clinical sleep apnea (that is, more than five apnea events of 10 seconds or more during an hour, or a total of 30 or more apnea events during a night) (4).

The consensus seems to be that a mild degree of apnea in otherwise healthy older people does not normally call for treatment, provided they feel well rested. However, a suspicion of sleep apnea should not be ignored. Drowsiness and loss of mental alertness are the worst enemies of the healthy senior, whose goal should be to remain as active and alert as possible. Apnea episodes contribute both to fragmentation of sleep and to a decrease in the oxygen content in the blood, which can lead to daytime drowsiness and loss of alertness. Seniors with other kinds of sleep disturbances, such as restless legs, show less daytime drowsiness (2). This suggests that sleep apnea may be a particularly significant cause of the daytime drowsiness seen in seniors.

If you are an older person who suspects that apnea is significantly disturbing your sleep and is causing drowsiness during the daytime, you may want to contact a sleep center for an interview and potential testing. If your snoring is disturbing your spouse or partner, but you are otherwise sleeping well and have a minimal amount of apnea, Somnoplasty may be effective (see Chapter 10).

Leg Movements During Sleep

Approximately 40 percent of older adults experience involuntary leg movements associated with sleep. In restless legs syndrome, a person has an uncomfortable or achy feeling and an urge to move the legs. This may interfere with falling asleep. Periodic leg movements (nocturnal myoclonus) are kicking motions that occur repeatedly during sleep. These may awaken the sleeper, but often they do not and are more disruptive to the bedmate. If you or your bedmate experiences either of these disorders, talk with a sleep specialist about possible treatment.

Medical Problems and Depression

Some less healthy older adults are bothered by medical problems that affect sleep (for example, pain from arthritis, respiratory problems, frequent urination, or leg cramps).

Depression is another condition that can affect sleep. The symptoms of depression often are attributed to "just getting old"—insomnia; pessimism; loss of interest; decreased energy; poor self-esteem; poor sexual functioning; increase in health complaints, such as constipation, back pain, abdominal pain, headache; social withdrawal; decreased appetite; and weight loss.

However, it is not true that aging inevitably leads to these difficulties. Healthy older adults who are not depressed do not routinely experience these symptoms. If depression is the cause of symptoms such as poor sleep, it is the depression that needs to be treated, not simply the symptoms.

The treatment of medical problems and depression that interfere with sleep is best carried out in consultation with a sleep specialist, as explained later, because some treatments can further interfere with sleep.

Getting a Good Night's Sleep

The most common sleep complaint among healthy older people is that they awaken numerous times during the night (1). People sometimes become worried about this pattern, and the worry itself—that they are "not getting a good night's sleep"—keeps them awake.

If you are a senior who is somewhat bothered by frequent awakenings during the night and drowsiness during the day, and you doubt that you have a serious sleep disorder, here are some helpful things that you can do for yourself.

1. Practice good "sleep hygiene." That is, try arranging your daytime life so that you promote good sleep:
   a. Eat regular meals.
   b. Get more exercise every day (but don't exercise right before bedtime).
   c. Go outside for a while every morning. Your biological clock needs light signals to regulate your sleep-wake cycle every day. Indoor light is not bright enough to work very well. Morning light, even on a cloudy day, can reset your sleep-wake rhythm and help you get better sleep.
   d. Eliminate daytime naps. They often are more the result of boredom than sleepiness. Find something active to do instead of napping.
   e. Plan evening activities—with friends or by yourself, either outside or in the home. Look forward to a full evening.
   f. Limit your caffeine intake (coffee, tea, cocoa, cola) and use alcohol moderately (alcohol actually interferes with sleep).
   g. Limit your fluid intake after 7 PM so that you will have less need to urinate during the night.

  h. Make yourself get out of bed and get dressed at a specific early hour every morning (say, 6:30 or 7 AM).

  i. Learn relaxation techniques to relieve the tension or worries that may be keeping you awake.

2. Reassure yourself that brief nighttime awakenings are normal and that you probably are actually getting enough sleep. This knowledge alone may release you from worrying about getting a good night's sleep. That, in turn, will probably let you sleep better.

3. If these suggestions are not effective, strongly consider seeking help.

If you try these suggestions in a disciplined way for several weeks and decide they are not helpful, make an appointment to discuss the problems with your doctor. If the symptoms are not resolved, ask your doctor about a referral to a sleep clinic.

If you have a medical problem that seems to be interfering with your sleep, check with a sleep specialist for ideas about a solution that will help you sleep better.

Sometimes the treatment for one medical problem may conflict with the treatment for another. For example, some drugs taken for heart problems can make sleep apnea worse. "Sleeping pills" nearly always make sleep apnea worse, as does alcohol. Barbiturates and some antidepressants have side effects that can affect sleep. A sleep specialist is likely to know more about these effects on sleep than your family doctor does, and the two of them should work together to find the most appropriate way of improving your night's sleep.

If sleep apnea is a moderate to serious problem or if you have other conditions, such as arrhythmias (irregular heart rhythms), congestive heart failure, or respiratory problems that are aggravated by sleep apnea, the sleep specialist may recommend treatment for your apnea. The type of treatment will depend on the kind of apnea and the severity of the problem (see Chapter 10 for treatment of sleep apnea).

◆ Summary

- Older people often get as much total sleep in 24 hours as young people do.
- However, the sleep of older people may be of poorer quality; that is, broken up by periods of wakefulness.
- Factors that can interfere with older people's sleep include sleep apnea, leg movement syndromes, pain, respiratory problems, frequent urination, medications, and depression.
- Seek help if you are persistently drowsy or if sleep disturbance is decreasing your quality of life.
- If you suspect sleep apnea, go to an accredited sleep center for an interview and possible testing.
- Mild sleep problems often can be solved by a program of good "sleep hygiene," as discussed in this chapter.

Finding a Sleep Specialist

Recognize trained sleep medicine professionals by their certification:

- Sleep medicine specialists have had advanced training in sleep medicine, have passed an examination, and are certified by the American Board of Sleep Medicine.
- Accredited sleep disorders centers have passed inspection by the American Academy of Sleep Medicine.
- Find a local accredited sleep disorders centers at www.aasmnet.org, click on *Patients and Public*, then click on *Find a Sleep Center*.
- Find a list of board certified sleep specialists at www.absm.org.

The State of the Art

If your car needs new brakes, you don't take it to a windshield shop. The same is true of sleep apnea.

Find an Expert

This is especially important to find a certified sleep specialist because sleep disorders medicine is a fairly new medical specialty, and few doctors are trained in the field. A survey of medical schools found that the average amount of time spent teaching about sleep was 20 minutes.

Because of managed care and financial arrangements with insurance companies, your doctor may want to send you to someone in his referral group who is not board certified in sleep medicine or does not even practice sleep medicine full time. Find out if your health plan is "capitated"—this means that every time your doctor orders a test it costs the clinic money. In a capitated setting, you are more likely to be denied care or to be offered potentially unproven or lower quality services. The doctor often may not consciously be trying to "save" money but may have been too ready to believe claims that some service is "cheaper" and "just as good." This may sometimes be true, but do you want to be the exception?

Most established specialties, such as pediatrics, obstetrics/gynecology, otolaryngology psychiatry, and so on, have their own departments in hospitals and medical schools. Medical students are taught by specialists in these fields, and they learn routines for diagnosis and treatment of illnesses in those areas. After medical school, doctors can spend several years in residency programs perfecting their skills in their chosen specialties.

But very few medical schools offer courses or programs in sleep disorders medicine. Consequently, very few doctors are trained to recognize and treat sleep disorders.

In the absence of established departments of sleep medicine in hospitals and medical schools, early sleep medicine specialists founded a professional organization to take on the role of setting the standards for professionalism in the field. Today the American Academy of Sleep Medicine (AASM, www.aasmnet.org) establishes the standards for the evaluation and treatment of sleep disorders, and provides accreditation of sleep disorders centers. The American Board of Sleep Medicine tests and certifies sleep medicine specialists.

The field of sleep disorders medicine is growing very rapidly. The AASM hopes the major medical schools will have programs on sleep disorders within a few years. However, until systematic sleep medicine training becomes part of the medical school curriculum, the public will have to look carefully to find a qualified sleep specialist.

Qualifications of a Sleep Specialist

The AASM defines a sleep specialist as "a physician who is . . . certified in the subspecialty of sleep medicine and specializes in the clinical assessment, physiological testing, diagnosis, management and prevention of sleep and circadian rhythm disorders."

The AASM membership consists of more than 6,000 physicians, researchers, and other health care professionals.

Look for a Board Certified Sleep Specialist

Doctors who are sleep medicine specialists have gone on after medical school to study sleep physiology through fellowship programs, graduate courses, or periods of practice at one of the major sleep disorders centers. A physician can earn a sleep specialist credential by passing the certification examination administered by the American Board of Sleep Medicine (ABSM). He becomes a board certified sleep specialist (BCSS). You can find a list of board-certified sleep specialists at the American Board of Sleep Medicine on the Internet at www.absm.org. Or you can call the American Board of Sleep Medicine (507-287-9819) and ask whether a particular doctor is certified in sleep medicine.

Some physicians who have trained in sleep medicine do not choose to become certified. Nevertheless, they may be well informed about sleep disorders. However, as in any medical specialty, a doctor's board certificate in sleep medicine assures you, the consumer, that the doctor has received special training and is qualified to carry out sleep testing and interpret the results of the tests. Finally, you should not start a treatment program for a sleep disorder before having a sleep study at an accredited sleep disorders clinic. This is particularly true if the treatment involves surgery. Read Chapters 8, 9, and 10, and seek a second opinion.

Standards for an Accredited Sleep Center

An accredited sleep center is one that has met the standards established by the AASM. As of summer 2007, there were more than 1,000 accredited sleep centers and laboratories in the United States. In addition, there were thousands of nonaccredited sleep laboratories nationwide. No one knows the exact number of nonaccredited sleep laboratories, but the AASM has received thousands of requests from sleep laboratories for information about earning accreditation.

A nonaccredited sleep laboratory may be good, but you have no way of knowing. Your family physician also is not likely to be intimately familiar with the details of quality sleep medicine and may just be referring you to someone in his group. However, a very wide range of quality exists, all the way down to some "street corner" sleep laboratories that are not reputable. The AASM has neither the funds, the staff, nor the mandate to "police" the entire field of sleep medicine beyond its own membership. And so far, no other organization or agency is keeping an eye on the quality of sleep testing that goes on in the non-AASM–accredited laboratories.

Find an Accredited Sleep Center

As a prudent consumer, if you want some assurance of professional standards in this new field, you may want to choose one of the sleep centers accredited by the AASM. You can find the accredited sleep disorders centers in your state on the Internet at www.aasmnet.org— click on *Patients and Public*, then click on *Find a Sleep Center*.

The standards for accreditation are broken down into two categories: full-service sleep centers and specialty laboratories.

Full-Service Sleep Centers

The requirements for accreditation for a full-service sleep center ensure that the center is able to deal professionally with the full range of sleep disorders. Here are the primary AASM requirements for a full-service sleep center:

- It must have an ABSM-accredited clinical polysomnographer (MD or PhD) on staff to read and interpret the results of sleep recordings.
- It must have a full-time physician with expertise in sleep physiology.

- It must have trained technicians to administer the sleep tests. Sleep centers are encouraged to have at least one technician who is accredited as a registered polysomnographic technologist.
- A private room must be provided for each patient, with sound, light, and temperature control and easy communication with the attendant.
- The facilities, testing procedures, and patient care must meet standards set by the ABSM.
- The sleep center must pass inspection by a two-member accreditation team every 5 years or it will lose its accreditation.

Specialty Laboratories

The standards for accreditation of a specialty laboratory are similar but tailored to a less extensive sleep testing role. Specialty laboratories usually deal primarily with pulmonary medicine (breathing disorders), and the diagnostic testing they do is mostly for sleep apnea rather than for the full range of sleep disorders.

The requirements for a specialty laboratory include the following:

- It must have at least one pulmonary specialist on staff.
- The staff must demonstrate knowledge of the practices and procedures of sleep disorders medicine.
- The physical surroundings, facilities, testing procedures, and patient care must meet ABSM standards similar to those for a full-service sleep center.

What to Do If You Are Denied Referral to a Qualified Sleep Specialist or Laboratory

Whenever you receive a denial or some sort of administrative delay in your health-care, it is best to remember a few important guidelines.

- First, if it is an emergency or the need for care is urgent, you need to proceed with getting the care you need and put off any consideration of insurance coverage, referrals, and administrative processes.
- Second, remain calm. You are not alone. The healthcare system is large and complicated. Sometimes it takes great patience to navigate it.
- Third, keep calling your insurance company and follow through with their processes and keep track of names, claim numbers, and other details.

In the case of sleep disorders, the three guidelines noted above apply as follows.

Fortunately, sleep problems usually do not require emergency attention, but if your need for sleep medicine care is urgent, you should move ahead and get that care. If office staff ask about a referral, billing issues, and so forth, explain the circumstances and that you will follow-up afterward. Get the information you have available to you such as health insurance policies and cards, doctor office and doctor visit information, bills, and any other relevant information.

Call the insurance company as soon as possible and explain your situation. Write down the name of the person you spoke to. (As silly as this sounds, it may make a difference later.) Get ready to tell your story many times to many people. (A speaker phone or other hands-free phone would be a very good investment before you do this. It is not unusual to be on the phone for a very long time.)

Be persistent. If you are given an answer you are not satisfied with, take the process to the next level of appeal. Often your primary care doctor can be helpful when appeals are necessary. Your doctor may be able to write a letter on your behalf or at least can forward medical records to your insurance company.

Don't Give Up and Just Go Anywhere!

If an appeal fails, write to your state insurance commissioner, whose office can be found by calling your state capital's government information number. All states have an individual or office that supervises insurance plans and health maintenance organizations (HMOs). Because of well-publicized abuses, insurance commissioners are very interested in identifying these types of problems.

How to Locate the Nearest Accredited Sleep Center and Sleep Specialist

The AASM will mail you a booklet listing the accredited sleep centers in the United States. Write to the AASM at the following address. Include a large, self-addressed, stamped envelope.

American Academy of Sleep Medicine
1610 14th Street NW, Suite 300
Rochester, MN 55901-2200
(507) 287-6006
www.aasmnet.org
American Board of Sleep Medicine
(507) 287-9819
www.absm.org

Choosing a CPAP System and a Durable Medical Equipment Company

- Ask your sleep center:
    - Which durable medical equipment (DME) providers that they recommend
    - Which continuous positive airway pressure (CPAP) brands and models they recommend
- Ask your insurance company which CPAP costs it will cover (purchase, rental, parts, service).
- When choosing a CPAP, consider comfort, quality, price, recommendations from a sleep center, and features that mesh with your lifestyle, such as size, shape, durability, adaptability, appearance, sound, availability of ramp setting and humidifier, and ability to run off a battery.
- Consider renting a CPAP in order to try different models
- If someone hands you a CPAP and tells you to go home and try it, run and find yourself a new sleep specialist!

Before you buy a car, you shop around. You may talk to several dealers, compare makes and models, and find out which dealers provide good customer service.

When you need a CPAP machine, you should do the same. You don't need to take forever to shop around. Your health is at stake, and you should start using CPAP as soon as possible after your doctor prescribes it. But some shopping can be worthwhile. After all, you will spend more time with your CPAP than you will with your car. The features of that CPAP machine and the homecare service you receive will become important to you.

Two Choices to Make

You will need to select the homecare company that will sell you the CPAP, and you will need to choose a CPAP machine and its attachments.

Start by asking questions at your sleep center.

1. Where can I obtain a CPAP machine? Companies that rent, sell, and service CPAPs are called durable medical equipment (DME) companies.
   - Ask your sleep center for a list of CPAP suppliers and DME companies in your area. Find out whether your sleep center is associated with a DME that supplies CPAP machines.
   - Ask your sleep center which DME companies they recommend, and why.
   - Ask if any local homecare companies have an unfavorable reputation.
   - Ask if the sleep center can put you in touch with other CPAP users. Go to an AWAKE meeting (for sleep apnea support groups, see Chapter 18 and the Appendix) and find out which homecare companies have given good service to other CPAP users. You may find that some local branches of a particular homecare company provide better service than others. Perhaps Company A has the best service in the north end of town, but on the south side the best service is from Company B.

2. What are my CPAP choices?
   - Which CPAPs does your sleep center think you should consider? Why?
   - What features do they suggest you look for (mask fit, size and shape of unit, durability, adaptability, appearance, and so on)?
   - What will your insurance pay for? Call your insurance company and ask them. This is important.

CASE STUDY

When Mr. Kennedy's sleep specialist prescribed a CPAP machine, Mr. Kennedy had no idea where to begin. His sleep center recommended that he call a DME company. He had never heard of DME companies. He didn't know that he could have chosen between several DMEs in his area and that different DMEs may carry different brands and models of CPAP machines. He didn't know that the features of CPAP units vary from one manufacturer to another.

He called the DME company that his sleep center recommended and got the first CPAP he saw. Fortunately, he was content with both decisions. However, if he had it to do over, Mr. Kennedy thinks he would ask more questions about other CPAP models and compare prices and services among several DME companies. (Many insurance providers now prefer that you rent for a month or two, which opens up some options to try different equipment.)

Choosing a DME Company

If you have never dealt with a DME company, you may not even be aware of their existence. DME companies rent, sell, and service health care equipment for use at home, including mechanical ventilators, oxygen, CPAP systems, and other home health care supplies.

You can ask your sleep center representative for a list of local DME companies, or you can find them listed in the Yellow Pages of your telephone book under Medical Equipment or Hospital Equipment and Supplies. The nationwide DME companies have branch offices throughout the country, but not all of them may serve your area.

The latest Internet fad is for DMEs to provide CPAP equipment online. You should be aware of several things about online CPAP unit purchases:

- You should not purchase your first CPAP unit online because you will need the benefit of a skilled respiratory therapist to get you started successfully.
- Not all online CPAP equipment purchases are covered by insurance. This is because the insurance companies understand that you will be much more likely to use and benefit from CPAP if you start out with the support, education, and other resources of a DME company with an office and respiratory therapists on staff.

Questions to Ask When Choosing a DME Provider

Select several DME providers and then visit their offices. See what they have to offer. Ask lots of questions. Take notes. Then compare.

1. What brands and models of CPAP do you supply? (A DME company may handle only one or two CPAP brands.)
2. How many CPAP setups do you do in a month?
3. Is the person who is going to set up my CPAP a licensed respiratory therapist or a respiratory care practitioner (as required in some states)?
4. Do you have a selection of different masks that I may try? (If the answer is no, find another DME provider right away!)
5. What services do you include in the price of a CPAP unit? Is there a charge every time I see the CPAP therapist? (Preferably, these visits are included in the price of the CPAP.)

The Ideal Service that You Should Receive from Your DME Company

Excellent support and service from your DME company may be the difference between successful treatment of your sleep disorder and a frustrating failure to improve. A good DME company will do everything it can to make sure you are successful with your CPAP and may have patient success rates twice as high as those of less supportive companies.

Getting Your CPAP Unit

You should have your prescription for a CPAP unit within a day or two after your CPAP titration night at the sleep center. Your first CPAP unit should be provided to you by a representative of the DME company you choose. The DME representative or respiratory therapist should be trained and able to set up your system properly, making sure the CPAP is set for the pressure and mode prescribed by your sleep specialist. He should instruct you about the use and care of the equipment and answer all of your questions.

Fitting the Mask

The DME representative should fit you with a CPAP mask under sleeping conditions—while you are lying down, and with the CPAP turned on. She should have an assortment of sizes and brands of mask available for you to try and should fit you with a mask that is comfortable on your face and does not leak. You should call your DME representative during the first week if you are not able to use your CPAP every night. She should continue to work closely with you for as many days or weeks as it takes for you to feel you have a comfortable, trouble-free CPAP setup. If the DME company is not helping you, call your sleep specialist.

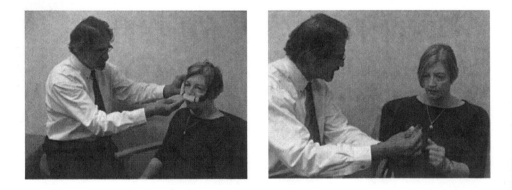

This well-trained CPAP technologist is making sure that the patient's new mask fits comfortably, and he is always available to help solve any CPAP problems that CPAP patients may encounter.

Future Service

Your DME should provide 1-or 2-day service in case of CPAP unit breakdown or emergency and the use of a "loaner" if you would be without your CPAP unit. Orders for new masks, filters, and other replacement parts probably will be mailed to you and should reach you within 2 or 3 days.

Many DME providers also offer a web site where you can order CPAP supplies with the supervision of a respiratory therapist. The therapist will review your order and help to make sure you are getting the correct replacement equipment. However, you should start on CPAP with a therapist *in person*, not with an online purchase.

Annual Service Visit

You should have your CPAP equipment serviced annually to make sure it is still working properly and delivering the correct pressure. You may have to ask for this service.

The Reality of DME Performance

In reality, many DME providers fall short of the ideal. Some DME companies deliver the equipment to your home, but the delivery person may not be trained to set up a CPAP unit (although many states now require that respiratory devices such as CPAP equipment be applied by a licensed medical person (for example, licensed respiratory therapist, RN, MD.). Some DME providers won't let you try on a variety of masks, claiming that would be unsanitary. This is cheap nonsense and a clear signal to immediately find another DME provider. Proper mask fitting is the most important CPAP service a DME provider should offer. Demand it!

Ask what services each DME will provide, and whether you have to pay extra for that service. If you're not satisfied, shop around.

You can always change companies if it turns out that you are unhappy with your DME company. Like a consumer buying a car or a dishwasher, you will need CPAP parts and service from time to time, and someday you will buy a replacement machine. A smart homecare provider should understand that you are free to take your business elsewhere and should be sensitive to your needs.

If your health care is provided by a health maintenance organization (HMO) or other insurance manager, it may have a contract with a particular DME provider that you will have to deal with. If that DME company won the contract by being the lowest bidder, service may be slim to none. Some DME providers even mail CPAPs to their HMO patients—sight unseen! HMO patients may have to be very assertive to get the service they deserve. You should report in writing any dissatisfaction with the performance of a DME company to your sleep center and to the medical director of your HMO, and you should continue to complain until you get the help you need or are permitted to use an alternative DME provider.

You may also choose to pay a little more and receive your CPAP equipment from an "out of network" DME—that is, a DME other than the one your HMO has contracted with.

In the *first two weeks* after you begin using your CPAP use, if you are not happy with your DME's service, complain immediately to your sleep center and find a new DME company.

Choosing a CPAP Unit

As with DME companies, be prepared to ask questions about CPAP options and make comparisons. Keep in mind the following:

1. You need a prescription to obtain a CPAP unit from a DME company. The prescription will tell what CPAP pressure you need and whether you need a type of CPAP machine with special features, such as a meter that records CPAP use.
2. Find out what CPAP unit costs your insurance will cover. Most insurance companies will not cover the cost of rental or purchase of a CPAP system unless a sleep study has been done to document the medical necessity for CPAP. Some require a specific prescription from the sleep specialist in order to pay for the more expensive machines, such as a bi-level, variable, or auto-adjusting "smart-PAP."
3. Consider renting for a month or two with an option to buy. Most insurance companies will pay for at least 1 month's rental, and Medicare requires a rent-to-purchase option.

Numerous makes and models of CPAP units are available (see examples in the illustrations in Chapter 10). CPAP technology is growing and changing so rapidly that we cannot describe specific makes or models (the information would be out of date by the time you read this book). The important thing is to compare features. Each model has unique features, so the choice may seem confusing at first. This is why it may be a good idea to rent and try out a model or two in the DME office before you purchase. Have the therapist connect you to the machine and turn it on, and allow you to breathe, paying attention to breathing comfort and the sound of the machine.

CPAP masks are sold separately from the CPAP unit. Many brands, styles, and sizes of masks are available (see illustrations in Chapter 10), and most masks can be used with most CPAP units.

The comfort and fit of the mask is so important that Chapter 18 is devoted entirely to mask fit and comfort.

Let's look at three major areas of comparison among CPAP units: quality, price, and special features.

CPAP Quality = Comfort, Reliability and Performance

You need a CPAP unit with:

1. Comfort. Newer machines with more advanced features are more comfortable for breathing.
2. Reliability. It must work properly all night, every night.
3. Performance. It must be capable of delivering a constant level of air pressure even when there is a leak around the mask.

In deciding on a brand, the least risky choice would be one of the top manufacturers. All have established track records for supplying high-quality products, parts, service, and support for their products. Currently, there are two leading manufacturers of CPAP equipment (see the Appendix for address, phone number, and web site):

- Respironics, Inc.
- ResMed Corp.

Respironics was the first manufacturer to make CPAP units commercially available. They have steadily improved and expanded their product lines while continuing to provide good service. As mentioned in Chapter 10, the company introduced a system in 1990 called BiPAP, with two variable-pressure settings, and have been leaders in the development of the auto-adjusting "smart-PAP." More recently, Respironics also introduced Cflex technology, which makes the pressure of the CPAP system easier to tolerate, especially for people who require higher pressure settings.

ResMed grew out of Baxter Healthcare, Inc., which in 1986 supported the commercial development of the original CPAP technology invented by Dr. Colin Sullivan in Australia. ResMed was the first manufacturer to incorporate several innovative features into CPAP—the universal power supply (1988); the delay timer, or "ramp" function (1989); and the Bubble Mask (1991).

These CPAP manufacturers have regional or local representatives who visit the sleep centers and the DME companies that carry their brand and train the employees in the proper use and maintenance of the equipment.

The staff of your sleep center has extensive experience with a variety of CPAP units. They may have several models that you can examine. You may want to ask them which manufacturer they prefer. Sleep centers usually choose manufacturers that they consider reliable suppliers of equipment and parts. Their choice may be a good recommendation.

Special Features

Each make and model of CPAP has features that make it unique. Your particular lifestyle, taste, or leisure activities may make one model more appealing to you than another.

CPAP masks and mask fit. This topic is so important that we have devoted a whole chapter to it (see Chapter 18).

CPAP sound. Are you or your bedmate sensitive to noise during sleep? Listen to the sound of several CPAP units under normal operating conditions; that is, while the CPAP is turned on, set at your prescribed pressure, and someone is wearing the mask and breathing normally. (It will sound different if it is turned on at a lower or higher pressure or is not being worn by someone.) Most CPAPs are so quiet that they produce only a gentle "white noise," which some people find actually lulls them to sleep. Listen to both the sound of the machine and the escaping air.

Ramp or not? Many CPAP units have a "ramp" feature, which starts the machine at a low air pressure and increases it slowly over a period of 5 to 45 minutes. Many people find that this gradual increase in air pressure allows them to go to sleep more easily, especially when they are first getting used to CPAP. The ramp feature sometimes can be part of the CPAP prescription. Ask your DME provider to show you how to use the ramp function.

CPAP unit size and shape might be important to you. Does the CPAP unit need to fit on your nightstand, or can it just sit on the floor? If you travel a lot, will it be easy to carry?

CPAP unit appearance. Is the appearance of the CPAP unit important to you? Do you care what it looks like sitting in your bedroom? Some models look more like medical devices, whereas others blend more naturally into the bedroom setting.

Humidifiers. Some people find that their nasal passages become stuffy or dry when using CPAP. A humidifier can really help to alleviate these problems. Some CPAP models have a built-in humidifier; some humidifiers heat the water, while others do not. If you experience nasal stuffiness or dryness on CPAP, you may want to ask your sleep specialist about a heated humidifier. Heated humidifiers are becoming almost commonplace because they add so much to the comfort of the CPAP user. A minor drawback to a humidifier is the need for cleanliness; you must dry the humidifier daily to prevent mold growth. The other drawback is cost, which can be $100 to $400 depending on whether it is heated. Insurance companies usually will pay for a humidifier if the doctor prescribes one because they know it improves patient comfort and therefore increases CPAP use.

Present and future lifestyle. You may want to give some thought to future activities— things you would enjoy doing once you have more energy. It is common for CPAP users to discover that soon they are able to be more active than they had been when they were slowed down by sleepiness or poor health. What would you like to do when you feel better? Take a trip to Europe? Invite that special person to spend the night? Go car camping, backpacking, or traveling across the country in a recreational vehicle (RV)? Charter a sailboat. . . . ? What features of a CPAP would enable you to fulfill that wish? If you are a car camper or boater or if you have an RV, what electric source will you want to use, and how easily can your CPAP be adapted? Many active CPAP users are looking forward to the advent of more battery-friendly models. One avid backpacker is lobbying for a mini-CPAP machine that could run on solar batteries attached to his hat! His dream recently moved closer to reality with the appearance if a little battery about the size of a paperback book that can run a CPAP all night. Who can even imagine the wonders that technology may find just around the next corner?

Prices

You may want to compare the prices for a particular CPAP model among several local DMEs. Ask what additional equipment and services they provide for that price. Contact your insurance company and find out how much they will pay for a CPAP unit. Will they pay for a Cflex-type or just a basic model? Will they pay for a heated humidifier? (Many will because it will improve the patient's comfort and willingness to use the CPAP.)

Currently, CPAP unit rentals are approximately $250 per month, and the purchase price for a basic CPAP model with a heater humidifier is about $2,000.

More complicated CPAP-type machines are more expensive. Bi-level and "smart" CPAPs units rent for about $350 per month and cost about $3,000.

You probably will have to purchase the mask and tubing separately (about $200 total) (these prices may vary across the country). The mask material tends to absorb oil from the skin and to become stiff, needing to be replaced about every 6 months, so that is a recurring expense. Some CPAP models have nonwashable air filters that need periodic replacement.

The price you pay should be "contracted" between your insurance company and the DME company. You will see this contracted price as the "allowed amount" on the explanation of your benefits. Your insurance company's customer service department can explain more about their coverage and the amount you may be responsible for paying.

You should have your DME company service your CPAP once a year, and at that time, you should actually replace your mask and tubing. Check with your insurance company to see if they will pay for these replacement parts.

Planning to Travel with a CPAP Unit? No Problem

1. By all means, do take your CPAP unit with you when you travel. Don't ruin your vacation or business trip with groggy days and sleepless nights.
2. Your CPAP equipment should always be in your carry-on luggage. Do not check a CPAP unit through as baggage—the risk of loss or damage is too high. Most CPAP units will fit into a carry-on bag and slide easily under an airplane seat. The slimmest new models even fit in a briefcase. Some manufacturers offer an attractive carrying case that probably is roomy enough to also hold a woman's nightgown and cosmetics. Your CPAP unit is "medical equipment" and should be permitted as a *third* carry-on by most airlines. Check with your airline if you need further information.
3. Durability. Select a CPAP unit that has, or can fit into, a durable case if you plan to travel with it.
4. Electrical adaptability. Electric supply involves 3 numbers: power (volts), frequency (cycles per second or Herz) and current (amperes or amps). U.S. electrical circuits operate at 110 volts and 60 Hz. Many European countries use 220 to 240 volts and 50 Hz. If you plan to travel outside the United States, find out whether your CPAP model can be plugged into or readily adapted for European circuits. The more advanced CPAP machines have internal automatic electric power converters that automatically sense the

correct voltage and frequency to use. If you often take long airplane flights, you may want to enquire about which CPAPs are approved for use on an airplane (110 V, 400 Hz). If you plan to travel overnight on European trains, be aware that they may not supply enough current (amps) to operate a CPAP. Most CPAP units require 1 or 1.5 amps.

To plug in your CPAP you will need the correct prong adapter for foreign countries. Luggage shops and travel catalogs sell a set of adapter plugs that will connect your CPAP to any plug in the world.

For travel "off the grid" (and as an alternative electric source at home in case of a power failure), there are batteries capable of running a CPAP all night. Deep cycle marine batteries work better than car batteries. A newer, small, lithium ion battery about the size of a paperback book is also available (see Appendix). This battery can be charged with the cigarette lighter in your car, making car camping with a CPAP unit easier than ever. However, if you intend to run your CPAP unit on a battery, check with the manufacturer to make sure it actually is able to do so. Some may not work or may require special adapters.

5. Airport security and Customs. Keep your CPAP unit easily accessible in your carry-on luggage so that security personnel can run a testing device over it. Usually that satisfies them: they are becoming quite familiar with CPAP machines.

6. Manufacturer's information. This can be useful in case of an equipment failure or emergency. Carry a manufacturer's brochure that describes your CPAP unit and includes phone numbers of people to contact in case of emergency. If you plan to travel in a foreign country, ask the manufacturer to send you a foreign language brochure and a company contact in that country.

7. CPAP unit travel accessory kit. Frequent travelers advise carrying the following, just in case: a three-prong plug, a 6-foot extension cord, an extra fuse, an extra of any small connectors between mask and tubing that might get lost or damaged, and adhesive or duct tape.

Do-It-Yourself CPAP and "Self-Titration"

An unfortunate trend in CPAP treatment is the "take it home and try it out" school of medical practice. Some people who are suspected of having sleep apnea—sometimes without even the simplest of sleep tests—are being handed CPAP machines and told to "just give it a try." What is wrong with this practice?

1. Do-it-yourself CPAP is trial-and-error medicine. The doctor is handing over his or her responsibility as diagnostician and healer to the patient, creating an unfair burden and usually an impossible task.

2. Do-it-yourself CPAP does not determine whether the patient has sleep apnea, another sleep disorder, or a medical condition that will remain untreated.

3. Do-it-yourself CPAP is unlikely to adequately treat the patient even if he does have sleep apnea. The patient has no idea what pressure to use. The pressure setting for CPAP should be custom-set ("titrated") for each patient in the sleep center in order to properly treat the sleep apnea without overtreating it. If a "self-titrated" patient is actually able to use the CPAP and actually does feel better, he still may not be adequately treated and the sleep apnea may continue to worsen.

4. There are hazards in both undertreatment and overtreatment with CPAP. Too low a pressure can leave the patient with sleep apnea symptoms that can result in the long-term effects of sleep apnea—high blood pressure, increased risk of stroke, heart attack, or heart failure. Too high a pressure can lead to poor acceptance of CPAP, poor sleep, increased mask fit problems, increased nasal problems, and in some severe cases cardiopulmonary problems due to central sleep apnea.

5. Do-it-yourself CPAP is a waste of money. It does not give the patient the support she needs to use CPAP regularly and successfully. Most do-it-yourself CPAP patients will remain untreated because the CPAP unit will stay unused in the patient's closet.

One reason we are seeing do-it-yourself CPAP is the increased pressure on HMOs and other medical providers to save money by treating patients as efficiently and inexpensively as possible, but this clearly is a short-sighted and false economy. If the patient remains improperly diagnosed and untreated, the long-term costs of untreated sleep apnea—automobile accidents, stroke, heart attack, heart failure—predictably are going to be much higher than if the patient had a sleep study and was properly titrated on CPAP in the first place.

What About Auto-titrating or "Smart" CPAP Units?

Another reason for do-it-yourself CPAP is the advent of "smarter" CPAP units. Smart CPAP units are the latest development in CPAP technology. Smart CPAP machines are supposed to be able to detect the patient's changing breathing patterns during the night and adjust the pressure to the patient's needs.

There is a misconception that anyone can send a patient home with a smart CPAP and properly diagnose and treat sleep apnea. In reality, this does not work well. For one reason, each manufacturer has a different method of determining how much pressure to use and when to change pressure. As a result, the comfort for the user varies considerably from one manufacturer to another, and some systems simply seem to work better for some patients than for others.

Initially, the smart CPAP units have been useful mainly in the sleep laboratory to aid in the diagnosis of sleep apnea and to determine the appropriate CPAP pressure setting for a patient. The computers in the smart CPAP units store data about the patient's breathing and the pressures used during the night, and those data can be downloaded to help the sleep specialist diagnose and prescribe treatment pressure for the patient.

Smart CPAP units may be appropriate for some carefully selected patients to take home for the night and return to the sleep laboratory for a diagnosis and a prescription for treatment. Smart CPAP units are best used under the direction of an experienced sleep specialist who is not simply trying to save money but actually knows that it would be highly effective in a particular case.

◆ Summary

- Ask your sleep center for a list of DME providers and CPAP units to consider.
- Ask your insurance agent which CPAP unit costs it will cover (purchase, rental, parts, service).
- When choosing a CPAP system, consider comfort, quality, price, recommendations from a sleep center, and unique features, such as size, shape, durability, adaptability, appearance, sound, and availability of ramp setting and humidifier.
- Consider renting a CPAP unit while you shop for a DME company and the CPAP model of your choice.
- When choosing a DME company, compare local reputation, the brands of CPAP units they sell, prices, and services.
- If someone hands you a CPAP unit and tells you to go home and try it, run for your life and find yourself a new sleep specialist.

The CPAP Mask: Getting Fit

- Everyone experiences a temporary adjustment period while getting used to CPAP.
- Be patient with yourself.
- Use the tips in this chapter.
- Don't hesitate to ask for help, and keep asking until you're satisfied.
- Support groups of other CPAP users can be extremely helpful.
- After a week, if you aren't sleeping all night with your CPAP, talk with your sleep specialist.

It's your first night at home with your CPAP unit. It's time to go to bed. You're a little anxious about this new equipment in your bedroom.

You're also kind of excited and hopeful. That morning in the sleep laboratory, after your first night of CPAP, you woke up feeling pretty good! If you can sleep like that every night, you'll be a new person!

Getting Started: 10 Steps

Who can remember 1everything the CPAP technician or respiratory therapist said about using this equipment? Because it's all so new, it is a good idea to get ready for that first night on CPAP sometime during the day, when you're not too tired. Then at bedtime, when you do feel tired and may not have a lot of patience left, everything will go more smoothly.

Here are 10 steps to a good night's CPAP.

1. Wash your face very well to remove all the skin oils. This will help the mask seal nicely against your skin and it will be less likely to leak. It also will make

the mask last longer. (Of course, you will wash the mask every morning as soon as you get up, so those skin oils don't sit on it all day.)

2. If your CPAP therapist has adjusted the headgear for you, it may not need adjustment now. If it has not been adjusted for you, attach the headgear to the mask now and slide it on over your head. Do some rough adjustments until you have a pretty good fit, then take it off for now. We'll fine-tune it later.

3. Place the CPAP unit near the head of the bed, making sure it is below the level of your head when you're lying in bed. It can be either on the floor, on a low table, or even in the closet if there is plenty of air circulation.

4. Attach the tubing to the CPAP unit and arrange it so it will lie or hang comfortably and not tug on your mask or fall off the bed. Some suggestions are to run it under your pillow; bring it up over the headboard; attach a cup hook to the wall above the bed or the headboard, slip a fat rubber band onto the tubing, and hook the rubber band onto the cup hook; bring the tubing under the blanket from the foot of the bed (this warms up the air a little). Many people use two lengths of tubing for more flexibility.

5. Attach the mask to the tubing. Turn on the CPAP unit. (Don't use the "ramp" until you have finished adjusting the fit of the mask at full pressure.)

6. Lie down on the bed, and slip the headgear with the mask over your head.

7. Pull the mask out from your face, then lower it to your face, to get any wrinkles out of the mask cushion. If you have a nasal pillow-type mask, make sure the pillows are in contact with your nostrils. Exhale through your mouth, and inhale through your nose, keeping your mouth closed. Congratulations! You're on CPAP!

8. Now adjust and fine-tune the headgear while you are lying down with the CPAP running. If the mask is leaking, first try pulling it out from your face and reseating it. If you need to adjust the tension on the headgear, do it a little at a time. The trick is not to get the headgear too tight, or (surprisingly) the mask may leak even more. Once you have the headgear adjusted so that the mask is not leaking, you can just slip it off and on over your head without unfastening it each time you remove the mask. Some masks have clips that disconnect the headgear from the mask, simplifying removal and putting it back on.

9. If you want to use the ramp feature, activate it now. Have it "ramp" up to full pressure in about 20 minutes. If you are not asleep in 20 minutes you can always activate the ramp again.

10. Now just lie there for awhile, relax, and breathe normally. Think about the beach, or imagine the clouds or your favorite restful place. If your mind wanders, keep returning to the most peaceful thoughts.

Improving Mask Fit and Eliminating Leaks

Causes of Leaks and Chafing

Getting a mask that fits properly is probably the biggest frustration most people encounter with CPAP. Air leakage around the mask and chafing of the bridge of the nose are two of the most common results of a poor fit. The reasons usually are:

1. The mask is the wrong size or shape.
2. The headgear is too tight or unevenly adjusted.

Your CPAP mask must fit securely and comfortably but not too tightly. Most people find that they need to experiment with the mask for a while to get a comfortable, leak-free fit.

Solutions to Poor Mask Fit

Your CPAP unit provider (also known as a durable medical equipment [DME] company) should be willing to try different sizes and brands of mask until you have an acceptable fit. If you experience leaks, chafing, or other problems, you need to immediately ask for help from your DME company. If the DME company representative doesn't respond, complain directly to your sleep specialist.

Always try on the masks with the CPAP machine running and attached to the mask, and while you are lying down in your normal sleeping position.

What steps can you take to get a leak-free fit? Tell your DME provider that you would like to:

1. Try a smaller mask. All masks come in at least two sizes, some in as many six!
2. Try a larger or wider mask.
3. Try several different brands of mask and several readjustments.
4. Try a "nasal pillows" type of mask; a smaller device with soft little cones (the experts call them "pillows") that fit up against the nostrils. Many people prefer these.

Masks Come In a Wide Variety to Choose From

Mask and headgear designs are constantly improving, so anything we write here will probably be out of date by the time you read it. But here is an example of the wide variety that should be available to you through a good DME provider. This is just a sampling, not a complete list or an endorsement of any particular product.

Respironics, Inc. (Pittsburgh, PA) makes a basic mask that has been the "standard" workhorse CPAP mask. Many people have been using that style of mask for 20 years and wouldn't change. It comes in several variations and eight sizes. Respironics also makes a gel-type mask, which feels rather neat and seals nicely against the face. It comes in four sizes. Their Optilife mini-mask fits up under the nose and has been redesigned with a light headgear that should make it easier to wear. Respironics also makes several different types of headgear that you might want to try. They publish a brochure and have a web site (see Appendix) that illustrate all of their masks and headgear.

ResMed Corp. (San Diego, CA) makes many interesting and comfortable masks. The Ultra Mirage is popular with many patients. It is small, light and comfortable. It comes in four sizes. It is sensitive to face oil and should be washed well every morning. The Swift mask is a nasal pillows–type mask. It comes in three sizes. ResMed makes a variety of headgear alternatives. Visit their web site (see Appendix) to see their latest gear.

Nellcor Puritan Bennett first developed the nasal pillows–type mask, which is a great favorite with many people, either for every-night use or as an alternative to the conventional mask. The tricks to a good fit are:

1. Get the right size (the cones come in six sizes).
2. Point them into your nostrils in the right direction and at the right angle.

Nellcor Puritan Bennett also makes "standard" style masks. They have pictures of all their many CPAP parts and accessories on their web site (see Appendix).

Most masks can be used with any CPAP machine. Exceptions: Respironics' Virtuoso machine and Aria LX machine set in alarm mode will not work with some masks. Also, some nasal pillows tend to leak at CPAP pressures above approximately 15.

Mask fit is a very individual thing. What fits one person's face and works well with his or her sleeping style may not work for another person. Listen to the suggestions of other people, but then try out the alternatives for yourself.

By testing the fit of several masks and fiddling with the adjustments, you will eventually hit on the right combination.

More Mask-Fitting Tricks

Overtightening the headgear is a common reason for chafing on the bridge of the nose. If your mask fits properly, you shouldn't have to tighten the headgear to the point of chafing.

Forehead adjustment. Several masks have different sizes of spacers to adjust the forehead support. This changes the tilt of the mask and increases or reduces the pressure of the mask on the bridge of the nose. Try wearing the mask a little looser and changing the forehead adjustment.

Cleanliness of both mask and skin is extremely important for discouraging leaks and skin irritation and prolonging the life of your mask. Wash your face every night before putting on the CPAP mask. If you have very oily skin, you may want to use a mild astringent, such as witch hazel, around the nose. The most important thing you can do to extend the life of your mask is to wash it with a mild, fragrance-free, oil-free soap as soon as you take it off in the morning. Let the mask air dry. Drying the mask by running the CPAP with the mask on the end of the tubing may dry out the mask and shorten its life.

In addition to cleanliness, masks work better if the contact between the cushion and skin is a bit tacky or sticky. Skin oil interferes with a good seal.

A *worn-out mask* will fit poorly, leak, and cause chafing. Most mask cushions are made of silicone, and silicone ages when exposed to air and to oil from the skin. A silicone mask should last for about 18 months, depending on the oiliness of your skin and how careful you are about cleanliness.

When the mask cushion becomes discolored or stretches out, it should be replaced immediately. Order a new mask as soon as the old one shows these signs or starts leaking, chafing, or fitting poorly. Skin abrasions from an ill-fitting mask are difficult to heal.

Sore spots. Once you have a sore spot, healing may be difficult because the mask will tend to irritate it every night. To prevent abrasion of the bridge of the nose and/or promote healing, look for wound-care products such as Restore (Hollister, Inc., Libertyville, IL) or DuoDERM (ConvaTec, Princeton, NJ). Ask your homecare representative. You also might try Second Skin (Spenco Medical Products, Waco, TX), a blister remedy that is sold in stores that sell running shoes or sports equipment. If you are using nasal pillows, you can lubricate the nose openings with a nonpetroleum product such as Ayr (B.F. Ascher and Company Inc., Lenexa, KS), a soothing saline gel that can help prevent irritation, or K-Y Jelly (Ortho Pharmaceutical Corp., Raritan, NJ). These products are available at most pharmacies. RoEzIt (LuSal Enterprises, Inc., Dallas, TX) is another nonpetroleum product that will help prevent irritation or dryness from nasal pillows.

Switch-offs. Some people switch back and forth between a mask and nasal pillows every few nights. They say this helps prevent irritation in the same places every night, and it gives them some variety.

There have been rare cases of eye irritation or infection either caused or aggravated by air escaping from around a poorly fitting mask. In the event of eye irritation, notify your sleep specialist. CPAP probably will have to be discontinued until the irritation clears up, or you may switch to a nasal pillows–type mask.

Other Common Mask-Wearing Problems

Claustrophobia and Mask Removal

Some people have trouble keeping the CPAP mask on all night. They may have a feeling of suffocation or claustrophobia, or they may unconsciously pull the mask off during sleep. This is quite common, and sometimes it is just a matter of getting used to the feeling of the mask.

If you continue to have either of these difficulties for more than a day or two, contact your DME provider or sleep specialist to discuss the matter. This problem sometimes is the result of nasal obstructions that are interfering with the CPAP. If this is the case, your sleep specialist will want to figure out the cause of the nasal obstruction; whether it is from allergies or another structural blockage. He may suggest treatment for the nasal obstruction to make CPAP more effective and comfortable for you.

The suffocating feeling sometimes is an anxiety about having the nose covered, and there are ways to work through it so that you can reach a point of being able to sleep quietly without being bothered by CPAP. Talk this over with your sleep specialist and try his or her suggestions (1).

Dry Mouth

Some people find that their mouth dries out during the night wearing CPAP. This usually results from sleeping with the mouth open. Sometimes it is because the nose is congested and the CPAP air cannot get through. Sometimes it is simply a habit. If you have dry mouth and a stuffy nose, you may want to discuss nasal obstructions with your sleep specialist. If your nose is stuffy, CPAP won't work for you. Another option is a full face mask, which covers both nose and mouth. If the open mouth is a sleeping habit, you may want to try using a chin strap to help keep your mouth closed. Keeping a glass of water by the bedside is another good idea.

Nasal Congestion, Dryness, or Runny Nose

Congestion, sneezing, dry nose, or very runny nose can be temporary responses of the lining of your nose as it becomes accustomed to the CPAP pressure. If you have these problems for more than a few weeks, you might want to talk to your sleep specialist about using a heated humidifier (see Chapter 17). A number of CPAP units come with a humidifier, and all can be used with a separate humidifier. An unheated humidifier is simpler and less expensive, but it requires a warm bedroom to be very effective. A heated humidifier is much more helpful, but it costs more and is a little more difficult to keep clean. Ask your DME provider which humidifiers they recommend. Your doctor probably will specifically have to prescribe a humidifier in order for your insurance to cover the cost.

If your nasal congestion is caused by allergies, ask your sleep specialist to recommend a decongestant. Some products are better for people with sleep apnea than others. You will most likely be advised to use the nasal decongestant for a maximum of three days.

Noise

The newer CPAP units are so much quieter than the vacuum cleaner–like earlier versions that noise almost isn't an issue anymore. If noise is a problem for you or your bedmate, there are many creative options. An obvious solution is earplugs. Try the kind that is shaped like soft, foam cylinders. They are sold in industrial safety stores and are quite comfortable. If you have had your CPAP unit sitting next to you on the floor or on a nightstand, try placing a piece of foam rubber under it, or moving it to the foot of your bed. If your bedroom closet is roomy and has good air circulation, you can run your CPAP unit there. Leave the door open a few inches to let in air. One ingenious CPAP user bracketed the machine to the ceiling of the room below the bedroom and ran the tubing up through a hole. These are the kinds of creative solutions you will hear about at AWAKE meetings from people who have been there (see below and Appendix).

All Night, Every Night—The Importance of Compliance

People fail to use their CPAP unit for many reasons. The most common cause of noncompliance usually is inadequate follow-up care—the user has not been properly introduced to CPAP, she does not receive proper follow-up help, or she does not understand that sleep apnea can cause major cardiovascular problems if CPAP is not used regularly.

Your Ticket to Enjoying Life

You should understand that CPAP is literally a lifesaver for you. You need to use CPAP every time you go to sleep—even for naps, even when you spend just one night away from home. Use CPAP because it offers you better health and longer life than you can expect if your sleep apnea is not treated. CPAP is your ticket to enjoying the things in life that are most important to you—instead of giving in to sleepiness, exhaustion, and poor health.

If you are having an equipment problem, your sleep center and your DME provider's staff should help you with troubleshooting. If your sleep center does not automatically offer the degree of continuing care you need, do not hesitate to request additional attention. You should receive whatever assistance you need to continue your CPAP treatment.

Acclimation to CPAP may take a couple of weeks. Stay calm, and be patient with yourself. Experiment. Don't give up! If you're not sleeping all night with your CPAP after a week, call your sleep specialist and ask for help. Ask and ask again, until you get it.

What If You Still Need Help?

If you:

- Don't have access to a sleep specialist.
- Don't have a well-staffed sleep center to turn to.
- Don't have a good homecare provider to help you.

CPAP Problems and Who to Call for Help

	Sleep Specialist	Sleep Center	DME Company	AWAKE/ Support Group
Mask fit, leaks, irritation	X Get help ASAP.			
Other day-to-day use problems (e.g., claustrophobia, insomnia, mask removal)	X			
CPAP equipment questions		X	X	X
CPAP repairs			X	
Learn about/ try different CPAP products, (size, shape, design, fit)		X	X	X
Do I *really* have to use CPAP *all* night? *Every* night?	X			
I don't feel any better. Is CPAP working for me?	X			
Solutions to medical problems: (allergy, infection, inflammation, medications)	X			
Weight loss and nutrition counseling	X Get referral to specialist.			

Then the next best thing is a support group—other people with sleep apnea. Here are some sources of support. The Appendix gives details about now to reach the following:

- AWAKE groups (local sleep apnea support groups) or workshops offered by a local sleep center.
- American Sleep Apnea Association (ASAA)
- American Academy of Sleep Medicine (AASM)
- Internet newsgroups and chat rooms offered by organizations with medical credentials, like the ASAA or AASM. Otherwise, take their information with a grain of salt.
- CPAP equipment manufacturers' local representatives

Other patients, possibly contacted through a support or AWAKE group, can be enormously helpful because they have been through the experience and can understand what you are dealing with. There is no problem that cannot be worked out. Solve the problem so that you can continue with the treatment and get on with your life. A CPAP unit does nobody any good if it spends the night unused in the closet.

Treatment Effectiveness

"I feel cured. Can I stop using CPAP?" Probably not. It is very common for people to report dramatic results from treatment. In fact, they often feel more improvement than has actually occurred. After uvulopalatopharyngoplasty (UPPP) surgery, a person may feel "completely cured" only to discover after retesting that he still has 50 percent of his or her sleep apnea. So don't assume that your sleep apnea has necessarily been thoroughly treated just because you feel better. Most important, don't assume that you can stop treatment because you feel better. Your sleep apnea will come back if you stop treatment.

Sleep apnea patients sometimes are asked to return to the sleep center by their sleep specialist after a specified period of treatment to be retested to verify that the treatment is effective. This is true not only for CPAP users but especially for sleep apnea patients who are being treated with medication, oral appliances, or surgery.

Another reason to be retested is if your treatment has not given you as much improvement as you had expected. A patient occasionally returns for retesting and the technicians find that the pressure on the CPAP unit was not properly set. Or the sleep specialist discovers a second sleep disorder that was missed or has developed since the initial sleep test. If you think you should be feeling better than you are, contact your sleep specialist.

Periodic retesting is important for all patients to make sure that the treatment remains effective over the years and that there is no return of the symptoms of sleep apnea. Most sleep centers will tell you when they want you to return for retesting. If yours does not tell you, ask what their policy is.

On Being a Pioneer

Today's CPAP users are medical pioneers. You are helping to teach the medical community how to recognize and treat sleep apnea. You are helping the sleep disorder centers to learn how to meet their patients' needs. You are helping the medical researchers and medical equipment manufacturers to invent better treatment methods.

The sleep disorders field is young in comparison with other medical specialties, and it still has some growing to do. The understanding of sleep apnea is not yet widespread throughout the medical community, but there are many well-informed doctors, many excellent sleep specialists, and many superb sleep centers in the United States and throughout the world.

Most important, today there are simple, effective treatments for sleep apnea that didn't exist even 2 years ago. There is hope now for many people who previously could not expect to see their sixtieth birthday.

You and your bed partner need to be assertive, well-informed consumers in this new field. Make sure your needs are met. Be patient, but not too patient. Be stubborn. Don't give up! Make sure your doctor listens to you. Seek the best-equipped, best-staffed sleep centers. Ask questions until you get answers. Learn the treatment options. Choose the conservative treatment over the risky one. Seek a second opinion on surgery. Find the experienced surgeons. Keep after your insurance company until they pay for your care. Demand service from your DME provider or switch to a competing company. Let them know if you are dissatisfied. And demand adequate follow-up care. It's your life.

◆ Summary

- Expect to go through a temporary adjustment period as you become accustomed to using CPAP. This experience is different for everyone.
- Patience, persistence, trial and error, asking questions, and demanding service are the keys to solving CPAP equipment problems.

Alternative Medicine and Sleep Apnea

CASE STUDY

Mr. Chambers was having trouble getting used to his continuous positive airway pressure (CPAP) machine. He was still waking up many times during the night and still feeling fatigued during the day. His sleep center scheduled him for a trial on BiPAP (Respironics, Inc., Pittsburgh, PA). With BiPAP, he slept through the night and felt refreshed the next morning. He arranged to buy a BiPAP unit and began using it nightly.

At about the same time, Mr. Chambers read an article that promoted magnetism as a treatment for a number of medical complaints, including fatigue. The article described the miraculous cures of several patients and claimed that these anecdotes "proved" the effectiveness of magnetism. The author of the article offered several magnetic products for sale.

Mr. Chambers wanted to feel better. He was impressed by the testimonials of the patients who had tried magnetism. He ordered several hundred dollars worth of magnetic bracelets, magnetic shoe inserts, and magnets to put in his mattress and pillow.

Today, Mr. Chambers feels more alert and energetic than ever before. He is convinced that magnetism has revitalized him.

A new field of medicine offers fertile ground for quackery. Unscrupulous people are quick to exploit people's hopes and fears. Claims of miracle cures for sleep apnea are already germinating among the "alternative" medical practitioners.

Who Can Diagnose Sleep Apnea?

Let's be clear on this. For an accurate diagnosis of sleep apnea, you need an overnight sleep test that follows standardized procedures. The results should be evaluated—and the treatment prescribed—by a well-trained, preferably accredited, sleep specialist.

Any alert doctor may suspect sleep apnea by looking at you, asking you if you snore, and performing a physical examination. But for an exact diagnosis and appropriate treatment, you need a sleep test.

Can Alternative Medicine Treat or Cure Sleep Apnea?

Alternative medicine cannot treat or cure sleep apnea. There is no sure cure yet for sleep apnea. There is effective treatment, but the sleep apnea will return if the treatment is stopped.

Sleep apnea is a complicated disorder, and the choice of the correct treatment depends on many factors, as explained in Chapter 7. The only known effective treatments for sleep apnea include one or more of the following:

1. CPAP
2. Weight loss for some people
3. Certain medications for some people
4. Certain surgeries for some people
5. A dental appliance for some people

Quack Detection: Rules of Thumb

Quacks are experts at appealing to our natural desire for a swift cure. Like most people with sleep apnea, Mr. Chambers didn't want to sleep with a CPAP machine. He was disappointed that his initial CPAP treatment hadn't worked as well as he had expected. He wanted a simple answer. He fell prey to a quack.

How can you recognize a quack? Who can you believe? And does it really matter if, like Mr. Chambers, you seem to feel better? Yes, it does matter, for two practical reasons:

1. Quackery is expensive. If you are on a limited budget, you can ill afford to spend your income on quack remedies.
2. Quackery can kill you, either directly with a dangerous product or indirectly by failing to treat a fatal disorder properly.

If you want to avoid the expense and risks of quackery, here are some rules of thumb.

1. Be skeptical. Question anything that seems too good to be true.
2. Look for the credentials of the person who is making the claims. Can he document any special training that qualifies him or her to dispense medical advice?
3. Question the research. Have the results been repeated and verified by other researchers? Have the results been reviewed by other scientists and then published in respected medical journals?

4. Follow the money. Who profits if you spend your money on this product or service? Is the cost reasonable, or is someone offering you a dime-store item for $50?

How does magnetism hold up to these rules of thumb?

1. Does it seem too good to be true that tiny, weak magnetic fields could abolish the effects of sleep apnea? Yes.
2. Does the "authority" selling this theory have medical credentials? No.
3. Does the research hold up? No. A Wisconsin sleep center measured sleep apnea symptoms with and without magnets and found "no benefit from magnetic therapy" (1).
4. Who profits from the sale of the magnets? The magnet merchants.

Did magnets revitalized Mr. Chambers? Or was his improvement more likely the result of his new BiPAP?

Alternative Medicine: What It Can and Cannot Do

With a few exceptions, most alternative medical practices are not harmful, provided they are not used as a substitute for good primary medical care.

If you would like to try alternative methods, at least be scientific about it. Discuss your ideas with your doctor, perform a controlled experiment yourself, and then be prepared to return to the sleep laboratory to find out whether there has been a measurable improvement in your sleep apnea.

Two Very Bad Decisions

One of the worst decisions you could make would be to stop using the treatment your sleep specialist prescribed while you try some new alternative. If you want to experiment with unconventional treatments (provided they are not harmful), at least continue to use your CPAP unit at the same time. If you stop using CPAP, your sleep apnea is guaranteed to return, and it will become worse over time.

The second bad decision would be to use an alternative practitioner as your primary or only doctor. Many alternative practitioners have limited medical training. They may fail to diagnose a serious disease (diabetes, cancer, heart condition) that could be fatal if it is not properly treated. If you must experiment with alternatives, do so in addition to good, regular, conventional medical care.

But Maybe This Really Is the Cure!

It's true—the cure for sleep apnea may indeed exist in some obscure alternative medical treatment. Many scientific discoveries originate outside the conventional establishment. The medical establishment is very slow to accept new ideas. Unconventional treatments are viewed with skepticism bordering on suspicion, and their proponents are often ostracized by the medical community.

Sleep disorders medicine itself is a perfect example of how long it takes to integrate a new concept into mainstream medicine. Sleep disorders research has been going on for more than 40 years, but sleep disorders medicine is only now beginning to be taught in medical schools. Yet this very skepticism is what guards the public from the quacks. New medicine has to prove itself through scientific method and peer review in the medical journals. This process prevents abuse and exploitation of the public by incompetent scientists, unscrupulous industries, and personal greed.

The system is not perfect. Some bad science is reported in the medical journals. Some good treatments take longer than they should to reach the patient. Progress seems slow, but continual advances are being made, and when the review process breaks down we are reminded of the value of deliberate skepticism and medical conservatism. For example, in the 1950s a poorly tested drug called thalidomide was recommended for pregnant women to combat morning sickness, and ended up causing severe birth defects.

If a sure cure for sleep apnea exists today, the medical community hasn't heard about it, much less had a chance to test it scientifically. Prudence suggests that we keep on using our CPAP units and remain patient and skeptical.

◆ Summary

- Rules of thumb for detecting medical quackery:
  - ○ Be skeptical.
  - ○ Ask for credentials.
  - ○ Know who profits and whether the product or service is worth the money.
  - ○ Learn whether the research followed scientific method.
- Keep using your CPAP if you decide to try alternative therapies.
- Do not use an alternative practitioner as your only or primary physician.

References

Chapter 1

1. D'Agostino RB, Grundy S, Sullivan LM, et al., for the CHD Risk Prediction Group. Validation of the Framingham Coronary Heart Disease Prediction Scores: Results of a multiple ethnic groups investigation. *Journal of the American Medical Association* 2001; 286:180–187.
2. Shahar E, Whitney CW, Redline, et al. Sleep-disordered breathing and cardiovascular disease: Cross sectional results of the Sleep Heart Health Study. *American Journal of Respiratory and Critical Care Medicine* 2001; 63:19–25.
3. Young T, Palta M, Dempsey J, et al. The occurrence of sleep-disordered breathing among middle-paged adults. *New England Journal of Medicine* 1993; 328(17):1230–1235.
4. Bixler EO, Vgontzas AN, Lin HM, et al. Prevalence of sleep-disordered breathing in women: effects of gender. *American Journal of Respiratory and Critical Care Medicine* 2001; 163:608–613.
5. Stoohs, R., L. Bingham, A. Itoi, C. Guilleminault, and W.C. Dement. Cross-sectional study of the prevalence of OSA in a population of long-haul truck drivers. Reported at the European Sleep Research Society meeting in Helsinki, 1992.

Chapter 2

1. Shahar E, Whitney CW, Redline S, et al. Sleep-disordered breathing and cardiovascular disease: cross sectional results of the Sleep Heart Health Study. *American Journal of Respiratory and Critical Care Medicine* 2001; 163: 19–25.
2. Partinen M, Palomaki H. Snoring and cerebral infarction. *Lancet* 1985; 2: 1325–1326.

3. Hung J, Whitford EG, Parsons RW, and Hillman DR. Association of sleep apnea with myocardial infarction in men. *Lancet* 1990; 336:261–264.

4. Watson R, Greenberg G, Deptula D. Neurophysiological deficits in sleep apnea (abstract). In *Sleep Research*, Vol. 14, p. 136. Chase M, ed. Los Angeles: UCLA Brain Information Service/Brain Research Institute, 1985.

5. Fairbanks D. Snoring: an overview. In *Snoring and Obstructive Sleep Apnea*. Fairbanks D, Fujita S, Ikematsu T, . Simmons FB, eds. New York: Raven, 1987.

6. Lavie P, Herer P, Hoffstein V. Obstructive sleep apnea syndrome as a risk factor for hypertension: population study. *British Medical Journal* 2000; 320:479–482.

7. Young T, Peppard P, Palta M, et al. Population-based study of sleep-disordered breathing as a risk factor for hypertension. *Archives of Internal Medicine* 1997; 57:1746–1752.

8. Shepard JW. Pathophysiology and medical therapy of sleep apnea. *Ear Nose Throat Journal* 1984; 63(5):198–212.

9. Strohl KP, Sullivan CE, Saunders NA. Sleep apnea syndromes. In *Sleep and Breathing*. Saunders NA, Sullivan CE, eds. Lung Biology in Health and Disease Series, Vol. 21. New York: Marcel Dekker, 1984.

10. Harper RM. Obstructive sleep apnea. In *Hypoxia, Exercise, and Altitude: Proceedings of the 3rd International Hypoxia Symposium*, pp. 97–105. Progress in Clinical and Biological Research Series, Vol. 136. New York: Liss, 1983.

11. Guilleminault C, Dement WC. Sleep apnea syndromes and related sleep disorders. In *Sleep Disorders: Diagnosis and Treatment*. Williams RL, Karacan I, eds. New York: Wiley, 1978.

12. Kohler U, Mayer J, Peter JH, Wichert PV. Cardiac arrhythmias accompanying sleep apnea activity (SAA) in patients with established sleep apnea and in general outpatients (abstract). In *Sleep Research*, Vol. 14, p. 179. Chase M, ed. Los Angeles: UCLA Brain Information Service/Brain Research Institute, 1985.

13. Jennum P, Schultz-Larsen K, Wildscheidtz G. Snoring as a medical risk factor. IV. Relation to lung function and hemoglobin concentration (abstract). In *Sleep Research*, Vol. 14, p. 173. Chase M, ed. Los Angeles: UCLA Brain Information Service/Brain Research Institute, 1985.

14. Podszus T, Mayer J, Penzel T, et al. Hemodynamics during sleep in patients with sleep apnea (abstract). In *Sleep Research*, Vol. 14, p. 198. Michael Chase M, ed. Los Angeles: UCLA Brain Information Service/Brain Research Institute, 1985.

15. Ryan CM, Usui K, Floras JS, et al. Effect of continuous positive airway pressure on ventricular ectopy in heart failure patients with obstructive sleep apnea. *Thorax* 2005 ; 60(9):781–785.

16. Kaneko Y, Floras JS, Usui K, et al. Cardiovascular effects of continuous positive airway pressure in patients with heart failure and obstructive sleep apnea. *New England Journal of Medicine* 2003; 348:1233–1241.

17. Mansfield DR, Gollogly NC, Kaye DM, et al. Controlled trial of continuous positive airway pressure in obstructive sleep apnea and heart failure. *American Journal of Respiratory and Critical Care Medicine* 2004; 169:361–366.

Chapter 3

1. Horstmann S, Hess CW, Bassetti C, et al. Sleepiness-related accidents in sleep apnea patients. *Sleep* 2000; 23(3):383–389.
2. AMA Council on Scientific Affairs. Report #1. American Medical Association, June 1996.
3. Aldrich MS. Automobile accidents in patients with sleep disorders. *Sleep* 1989; 12(6):487–494.
4. Powell NB, Schechtman KB, Riley RW, et al. The road to danger: the comparative risks of driving while sleepy. *Laryngoscope* 2001; 111:887–893.
5. Hartenbaum N, Collop N, Rosen IM, et al. SA & Commercial Motor Vehicle Operators: Statement from the Joint Task Force of the American College of Chest Physicians, American College of Occupational and Environmental Medicine, and the National Sleep Foundation. *Journal of Occupational and Environmental Medicine* 48(9 Suppl), 2006.
6. Young T, Blustein J, Finn L, Palta M. Sleep-disordered breathing and motor vehicle accidents in a population-based sample of employed adults. *Sleep* 1997; 20(8):608–613.
7. Stoohs R, Bingham L, Itoi A, et al. Cross-sectional study of the prevalence of OSA in a population of long-haul truck drivers. Reported at the European Sleep Research Society meeting in Helsinki, 1992.
8. Pack AI, Dinges D, Maisolin G. *A Study of Prevalenceo Of Sleep Apnea Among Commercial Truck Drivers.* Federal Motor Carrier Safety Administration Publication No. DOT-RT-02-030. Washington, DC, 2002.

Chapter 4

1. Naegele B, Thouvard V, Pepin J-L, et al. Deficits of cognitive executive function in patients with sleep apnea syndrome. *Sleep* 1995; 18(1):43–52.
2. Fairbanks D. Snoring: an overview. In *Snoring and Obstructive Sleep Apnea.* Fairbanks D, Fujita S, Ikematsu T, Simmons FB, eds. New York: Raven, 1987.
3. Beebe DW, Gozal D. Obstructive sleep apnea and the prefrontal cortex: towards a comprehensive model linking nocturnal upper airway obstruction to daytime cognitive and behavioral deficits. *Journal of Sleep Research* 2002; 11:1-16.
4. Cartwright R, Knight S. Silent partners: the wives of sleep apneic patients. *Sleep* 1987; 10(3):244–248.

Chapter 5

1. Guilleminault C, Lugaresi E. *Sleep/Wake Disorders: Natural History, Epidemiology, and Long-Term Evolution.* New York: Raven, 1983.

2. Lavie P, Rubin AE. Effects of nasal occlusion on respiration in sleep: evidence of inheritability of sleep apnea proneness. *Acta Oto-laryngologia* (Stockh) 1984; 97(1–2):127–130.

3. Young, T, Palta M, Dempsey J, et al. The occurrence of sleep-disordered breathing among middle-aged adults. *N Engl J Med* 1993; 328(17):1230–1235.

4. Dement WC. *Some Must Watch While Some Must Sleep*. San Francisco: Freeman, 1972.

5. Orr WC. Utilization of polysomnography in the assessment of sleep disorders. *Medical Clinics of North America* 1985; 69(6):1153–1167.

6. Lavie P. Sleep apnea in industrial workers. In *Sleep/Wake Disorders: Natural History, Epidemiology, and Long-Term Evolution*. New York: Raven, 1983.

7. Hales D. *The Complete Book of Sleep: How Your Nights Affect Your Days Reading*. North Reading, Mass.: Addison-Wesley, 1981.

Chapter 6

1. Dement WC. *Some Must Watch While Some Must Sleep*. San Francisco: Freeman, 1972.

2. Randazzo AC, Schweitzer PK, Walsh JK. Cognitive function following 3 nights of sleep restriction in children 10–14. *Sleep* 1998; 21(Suppl):249.

3. Johnson D, Thorne D, Rowland L, et al. The effects of partial sleep deprivation on psychomotor vigilance. *Sleep* 1998; 21(Suppl):204.

4. Dawson D, Reid K. Fatigue, alcohol and performance impairment. *Nature* 1997; 388:235.

5. Shepard JW. Pathophysiology and medical therapy of sleep apnea. Ear Nose Throat Journal 1984; 63(5):198–212.

6. Lugaresi E, Mondini S, Zucconi M, et al. Staging of heavy snorers' disease: a proposal. In Proceedings of the 4th International Congress of Sleep Research Satellite Symposium (Bologna). *Bulletin Européen de Physiopathologie Respiratoire* 1983; 19(6):590–594.

Chapter 7

1. Jamieson A, Guilleminault C, Partinen M, Quera–Salva MA. Obstructive sleep apnea patients have craniomandibular abnormalities. Sleep 1986; 9(4):469–477.

2. Shepard JW. Pathophysiology and medical therapy of sleep apnea. *Ear Nose Throat Journal* 1984; 63(5):198–212.

3. Guilleminault C. Stanford Sleep Disorders Center, Stanford, California. Interview, March 28, 1986.

4. Sin D, Logan AG, Fitzgerald FS, et al. Effects of continuous positive airway pressure on cardiovascular outcomes in heart failure patients with and without Cheyne-Stokes respiration. *Circulation* 2002; 102:61–66.

Chapter 8

1. Dement W. Statement on the Findings and Recommendations of the National Commission on Sleep Disorders Research, Field hearing before U.S. Senate Appropriations Committee, Portland, Oregon, November 4, 1992.

Chapter 9

1. Standards of Practice Committee of the American Sleep Disorders Association. Practice parameters for the use of portable recording in the assessment of obstructive sleep apnea. *Sleep* 1994; 17(4):372–377.
2. American Sleep Disorders Association Standards of Practice Committee. Practice parameters for the indications for polysomnography and related procedures. *Sleep* 1997; 20(6):406–422.

Chapter 10

1. Sullivan CE, Berthon–Jones M, Issa FG, and Eves L. Reversal of obstructive sleep apnoea by continuous positive airway pressure applied through the nares. *Lancet* 1981; 1(8225):862–865.
2. Issa FG, Sullivan.CE. Reversal of central apnea using nasal CPAP. *Chest* 1986; 90(2):165–176.
3. Sanders MH, Gruendl CA, Rogers RM. Patient compliance with nasal CPAP therapy for sleep apnea. *Chest* 1986; 90(3):330–333.
4. Soll BA., George PT. Treatment of obstructive sleep apnea with a nocturnal airway-patency appliance. *New England Journal of Medicine* 1985; 313(6):386, 387.
5. Andrews JN, Guilleminault C, Holdaway RA. Retaining devices and mandibular positioning appliances. In Proceedings of the 4th International Congress of Sleep Research Satellite Symposium (Bologna). *Bulletin Européen de Physiopathologie Respiratoir* 1983; 19(6):611.
6. Avidan, AY, Golish JA, Dinner DS, et al. The mandibular advancement device for the treatment of obstructive sleep apnea. Abstract C100.K1. *Sleep* 1999; 22(Suppl 1).
7. Parker JA, Kathwalla S, Ravenscraft S, et al. A prospective study evaluating the effectiveness of a mandibular repositioning appliance (PM Positioner) for the treatment of moderate obstructive sleep apnea. Abstract C376.K1. *Sleep* 1999; 22(Suppl 1).
8. Barbosa RC, Aloe FS, Taveres ST, Silva AB. Oral appliance treatment: PSG results in 16 mild to severe OSAS subjects. Abstract C502.J. Sleep 1999; 22(Suppl 1).
9. American Sleep Disorders Association. Standards of Practice Committee. Practice parameters for the treatment of snoring and obstructive sleep apnea with oral appliances. *Sleep* 1995; 18(6):511–513.

10. Rose EC, Barthlen GM, Staats R, Jonas IE. Therapeutic efficacy of an oral appliance in the treatment of obstructive sleep apnea: a 2-year follow-up. *American Journal of Orthodontics and Dentofacial Orthopedics* 2002;121(3):273–79.

11. Cartwright RD, Samelson CF. Effects of a non-surgical treatment for obstructive sleep apnea—the tongue-retaining device. *Journal of the American Medical Association* 1982; 248(6): 705–709.

12. Cartwright RD. Predicting response to the tongue retaining device for sleep apnea syndrome. *Archives of Oto-laryngolgia* 1985; 111:385–388.

13. Moore RW. OPAP: A new approach to the management of obstructive sleep apnea. *Functional Orthodontia* 2000; 17(1):29–30.

14. Yousefian J, Trimble D, and Folkman G. A new look at the treatment of Class II Division 2 malocclusions. *American Journal of Orthodontics and Dentofacial Orthopedics* 2006; 130(6): 771–778.

15. Gotfried MH, Quan SF. Obstructive sleep apnea—pathogenesis and treatment. *Lung* 1984;162:1–13.

16. Brownell LG, Perez-Padilla R, West P, Kryger MH. The role of protriptyline in obstructive sleep apnea. In Proceedings of the 4th International Congress of Sleep Research Satellite Symposium (Bologna). *Bulletin Européen de Physiopathologie Respiratoire* 1983; 19(6):621–624.

17. Guilleminault C, Mondini S. Need for multi-diagnostic approaches before considering treatment in obstructive sleep apnea. In Proceedings of the 4th International Congress of Sleep Research Satellite Symposium (Bologna). *Bulletin Européen de Physiopathologie Respiratoire* 1983; 19(6):583–589.

18. Guilleminault C, Dement WC. Sleep apnea syndromes and related sleep disorders. In *Sleep Disorders: Diagnosis and Treatment*. Williams RL, Karacan I, eds. New York: Wiley, 1978.

19. Smith PL, Haponik EF, Allen RP, Bleecker ER. The effects of protriptyline in sleep-disordered breathing. *American Review of Respiratory Diseases* 1983; 127:8–13.

20. Colman M.F. Limitations, pitfalls, and risk management in palatopharyngoplasty. In *Snoring and Obstructive Sleep Apnea*. Fairbanks D, Fujita S, Ikematsu T, Simmons FB, eds. New York: Raven, 1987.

21. Thawley SE. Surgical treatment of obstructive sleep apnea. *Medical Clinics of North America* 1985; 69(6):1337–1357.

22. Conway W, Fujita S, Zorick F, et et al. Uvulopalatopharyngoplasty: one-year follow-up. *Chest* 1985; 88(3):385–387.

23. Guilleminault C, Hayes B, Smith L, Simmons FB. Palatopharyngoplasty and obstructive sleep apnea syndrome. In Proceedings of the 4th International Congress of Sleep Research Satellite Symposium (Bologna). *Bulletin Européen de Physiopathologie Respiratoire* 1983; 19(6):595–599.

24. Katsantonis GP, Walsh JK, Schweitzer PK, Friedman WH. Further evaluation of uvulopalatopharyngoplasty in the treatment of obstructive sleep apnea syndrome. *Otolaryngology Head and Neck Surgery* 1985; 93(2):244–250.

25. Fujita S, Conway WA, Zorick FJ, et al. Evaluation of the effectiveness of uvulopalatopharyngoplasty. *Laryngoscope* 1985; 95:70–74.

26. Riley R, Guilleminault , Powell N, Simmons FB. Palatopharyngoplasty failure, cephalometric roentgenograms, and obstructive sleep apnea. *Otolaryngology Head and Neck Surgery* 1985; 93(2):240–243.

27. Riley R, Guilleminault C, Herran J, Powell N. Cephalometric analyses and flow-volume loops in obstructive sleep apnea patients. *Sleep* 1983; 6(4):303–311.

28. Jamieson A, Guilleminault C, Partinen M, Quera–Salva MA. Obstructive sleep apnea patients have craniomandibular abnormalities. *Sleep* 1986; 9(4): 469–477.

29. Moran WB Jr. Obstructive sleep apnea: diagnosis by history, physical exam, and special studies. In *Snoring and Obstructive Sleep Apnea*. Fairbanks D, Fujita S, Ikematsu T, Simmons FB, eds. New York: Raven, 1987.

30. Shepard JW Jr, Gefter WB, Guilleminault C, et al. Evaluation of the upper airway in patients with obstructive sleep apnea. *Sleep* 1991; 14(4):361–371.

31. Penek J. Laser-assisted uvulopalatoplasty: the cart before the horse. *Chest* 1995; 107(1):1–3.

32. American Sleep Disorders Association. Standards of Practice Committee. Practice parameters for the use of laser-assisted uvulopalatoplasty. *Sleep* 1994; 17(8):744–748.

33. Wareing MJ, Callanan VP, Mitchell DB. Laser assisted uvulopalatoplasty: six and eighteen month results. *Journal of Laryngology and Otology* 1998; 112(7):639–641.

34. Powell NB, Riley RW, Troell RJ, et al. Radiofrequency volumetric tissue reduction of the palate in subjects with sleep-disordered breathing. *Chest* 1998; 113(5):1163–1174.

35. Powell NB, Riley RW. Radiofrequency tongue base reduction in sleep disordered breathing: a pilot study. *Otolaryngology Head and Neck Surgery* 1998; 119(2):5.

36. Fujita S, Woodson T, Clark JL, Wittig R. Laser midline glossectomy as a treatment for obstructive sleep apnea. *Laryngoscope* 1991; 101:805–809.

37. Mickelson SA, Rosenthal L. Midline glossectomy and epiglottidectomy for obstructive sleep apnea syndrome. *Laryngoscope* 1997; 107:614–619.

38. Walker RP. Palatal implants: a new approach for the treatment of obstructive sleep apnea. *Otolaryngology Head and Neck Surgery* 2006; 135(4): 549–554.

39. Friedman M. Palatal stiffening after failed uvulopalatopharyngoplasty with the Pillar Implant System. *Laryngoscope* 2006; 116(11):1956–1961.

40. Riley RW, Powell NB, Guilleminault C. Obstructive sleep apnea syndrome: a surgical protocol for dynamic upper airway reconstruction. *J Oral Maxillofac Surg* 1993; 51(7):742–747.

41. Riley R, Guilleminault C, Powell N, Derman S. Mandibular osteotomy and hyoid bone advancement for obstructive sleep apnea: a case report. *Sleep* 1984; 7(1):79–82.

42. Powell N, Guilleminault C, Riley R, Smith L. Mandibular advancement and obstructive sleep apnea syndrome. In Proceedings of the 4th International Congress of Sleep Research Satellite Symposium (Bologna). *Bulletin Européen de Physiopathologie Respiratoire* 1983; 19(6):607–610.

43. Guilleminault C, Simmons FB, Motta J, et al. Obstructive sleep apnea syndrome and tracheostomy: long-term follow-up experience. *Arch Intern Med* 1981; 141:985–988.

44. Lubin MF, Walker HK, Smith RB III, eds. *Medical Management of the Surgical Patient.* 2nd ed. London: Butterworths, 1988.

45. Charuzi I, Ovnat A, Peiser J, Saltz H, et al. The effect of surgical weight reduction on sleep quality in obesity-related sleep apnea syndrome. *Surgery* 1985; 97(5):535–538.

46. Buchwald H. Bariatric surgery for morbid obesity: Health implications for patients, health professionals, and third-party payers. *Journal of the American College of Surgeons* 2005; 200(4):

47. Spivak H, Hewitt MF, Onn A, et al. Weight loss and improvement of obesity-related illness in 500 U.S. patients following laparoscopic adjustable gastric banding procedure. *American Journal of Surgery* 2005; 189(1):

48. White DP, Zwillich CW, Pickett CK, et al. Central sleep apnea: improvement with acetazolamide therapy. *Archive of Internal Medicine* 1982; 142:1816–1819.

49. Whyte KF, Gould GA, Airlie MAA, et al. Role of protriptyline and acetazolamide in sleep apnea/hypopnea syndrome. *Sleep* 1988; 11(5):463–472.

50. Shore ET, Millman RP. Central sleep apnea and acetazolamide therapy (letter). *Archives of Internal Medicine* 1983; 143:1278, 1280.

51. Guilleminault C, van den Hoed J, Mitler MM. Clinical overview of the sleep apnea syndromes. In *Sleep Apnea Syndromes*, Kroc Foundation Series, Vol. 11. Guilleminault C, Dement WC, eds. New York: Liss, 1978.

52. Douglas NJ, Connaughton JJ, Morgan AD, et al. Effect of almitrine on nocturnal hypoxaemia in chronic bronchitis and emphysema, and in patients with central sleep apnea. In Proceedings of the 4th International Congress of Sleep Research Satellite Symposium (Bologna). *Bulletin Européen de Physiopathologie Respiratoire* 1983; 19(6):631.

53. Krieger J, P. Mangin P, Kurtz D. Almitrine and sleep apnea. *Lancet* 1982; 9(8291):210.

54. White DP. Central sleep apnea. *Medical Clinic of North America* 1985; 69(6):1205–1219.

55. Meisner H, Schober JG, Struck E, et al. Phrenic nerve pacing for the treatment of central hypoventilation syndrome—state of the art and case report. *Thoracic and Cardiovascular Surgeon* 1983; 31:21–25.

56. Brouillette RT, Ilbawi MN, Hunt CE. Phrenic nerve pacing in infants and children: a review of experience and report on the usefulness of phrenic nerve stimulation studies. *Journal of Pediatrics* 1983; 102(1):32–39.

57. Glenn WWL, Phelps M, Gersten LM. Diaphragm pacing in the management of central alveolar hypoventilation. In *Sleep Apnea Syndromes*, Kroc Foundation Series, Vol. 11. Guilleminault C, Dement WC, eds. New York: Liss, 1978.

Chapter 11

1. Brooks B, Cistulli PA, Borkman M, et al. Obstructive sleep apnea in obese non–insulin-dependent diabetic patients: effect of continuous positive airway pressure treatment on insulin responsiveness. *Journal of Clinical Endocrinology & Metabolism* 1994; 79(6):11681–11685.

2. Wilcox I, Grunstein RR, Hedner, et al. Effect of nasal continuous positive airway pressure during sleep in 24-hour blood pressure in obstructive *sleep* apnea. Sleep 1993; 16:539–544.

3. Cooper BG, White JES, Ashworth L, et al. Hormonal and metabolic profiles in subjects with obstructive sleep apnea syndrome and the acute effects of nasal continuous positive airway pressure (CPAP) treatment. *Sleep* 1995; 18(3):172–179.

4. Waldhorn RE. Cardiopulmonary consequences of obstructive sleep apnea. In *Snoring and Obstructive Sleep Apnea*. Fairbanks D, Fujita S, Ikematsu T, Simmons FB, eds. New York: Raven, 1987.

5. Kryger MH. Sleep apnea: from the needles of Dionysius to continuous positive airway pressure. *Archives of Internal Medicine* 1983; 143(12):2301–2303.

6. Lavie P. Nothing new under the moon: historical accounts of sleep apnea syndrome. *Arcives of Internal Medicine* 1984; 144(10):2025–2028.

7. Gastaut H, Tassinari CA, Duron B. Polygraphic study of the episodic diurnal and nocturnal (hypnic and respiratory) manifestations of the Pickwick syndrome. *Brain Res* 1966; 2:167–186.

8. Jung R, Kuhlo W. Neurophysiological studies of abnormal night sleep in the Pickwickian syndrome. *Progress in Brain Research: Sleep Mechanisms* 1965; 18:140–159.

9. Charuzi I, Ovnat A, Peiser J, et al. The effect of surgical weight reduction on sleep quality in obesity-related sleep apnea syndrome. *Surgery* 1985; 97(5):535–538.

10. Sidney BC, Robin ED, Whaley RD, Bikelman AG. Extreme obesity associated with alveolar hypoventilation—a Pickwickian syndrome. *American Journal of Medicine* 1956; 21:811–818.

11. Sullivan CE, Berthon-Jones M, Issa FG. Remission of severe obesity-hypoventilation syndrome after short-term treatment during sleep with nasal continuous positive airway pressure. *American Review of Respiratory Diseases* 1983; 128(1):177–181.

Chapter 12

1. Hodgman JE, Hoppenbrouwers T. Cardiorespiratory behavior in infants at increased epidemiological risk for SIDS. In *Sudden Infant Death Syndrome: Proceedings of*

the 1982 *International Research Conference* (Baltimore). Tildon JT, Roeder LM, Steinschneider A, eds. New York: Academic, 1983.

2. Albani M, Bentele KHP, Budde C, Schulte FJ. Infant sleep apnea profile: preterm vs. term infants. *European Journal of Pediatrics* 1985; 143(4):261–268.

3. Stoddard RA, Auxier P. Predischarge evaluation for apnea and bradycardia in premature infants. *Pediatric Pulmonology* 1998; 26:448.

4. Guilleminault C, ed. Sleep apnea in the full-term infant. In Sleep and Its *Disorders in Children*. New York: Raven, 1987.

5. McNamara F, Sullivan CE. Evolution of sleep-disordered breathing and sleep in infants. *Journal of Paediatrics and Child Health* 1998; 34(1):37–43.

6. Limerick, The Countess of. Greetings. In *Sudden Infant Death Syndrome: Proceedings of the 1982 International Research Conference* (Baltimore). Tildon JT, Roeder M, Steinschneider A, eds. New York: Academic, 1983.

7. Kohlendorfer U, Kiechl S, Sperl W. Sudden infant death syndrome: risk factor profiles for distinct subgroups. *American Journal of Epidemiologu* 1998; 147(10):960–968.

8. National Institutes of Health Consensus Development Conference on Infantile Apnea and Home Monitoring. *Pediatrics* 1987; 79:292–299.

9. American Academy of Pediatrics. AAP Task Force on Infant Positioning and SIDS. *Pediatrics* 1992; 89(6 Pt 1):1120–1126.

10. Golding J, Limerick S, Macfarlane A. *Sudden Infant Death: Patterns, Puzzles, and Problems*. Seattle: University of Washington Press, 1985.

11. Guilleminault C, Robinson A. Developmental aspects of sleep and breathing. *Current Opinion in Pulmonary Medicine* 1996; 2(6):492–9. Review.

12. Downey R III, Perkin M, MacQuarrie J. Nasal CPAP use in children with obstructive sleep apnea under 2 years of age. *Pediatric Pulmonology* 1998; 26:443.

13. Marcus CL, Carroll JL,. Koerner CB, et al. Determinants of growth in children with the obstructive sleep apnea syndrome. *Journal of Pediatrics* 1994; 124(4):556–562.

Chapter 13

1. Rosen CL. Obstructive sleep apnea syndrome in children: controversies in diagnosis and treatment. *Pediatric Clinics of North America* 2004; 51(1): 153–167.

2. Chervin RD, Archbold KH, Dillon JE, et al. Inattention, hyperactivity, and symptoms of sleep-disordered breathing. Pediatrics 2002; 109(3):449–456.

3. Gozal D, Pope DW Jr. Snoring during early childhood and academic performance at ages thirteen to fourteen years. *Pediatrics* 2001; 107(6):1394–1399.

4. Stradling JR, Thomas G,. Warley ARH, et al. Effect of adenotonsillectomy on nocturnal hypoxaemia, sleep disturbance, and symptoms in snoring children. *Lancet* 1990; 335:249–53.

5. Gozal D. Sleep disordered breathing and school performance in children. *Pediatrics* 1998; 102(3):616–620.

6. American Academy of Pediatrics, Section on Pediatric Pulmonology, Subcommittee on Obstructive Sleep Apnea Syndrome. Clinical practice guideline: diagnosis and management of childhood obstructive sleep apnea syndrome. *Pediatrics* 2002; 109(4):704–712.

7. Ferber R. *Solve Your Child's Sleep Problems.* New York: Simon & Schuster, 1985.

8. Guilleminault C, Korobkin R, Winkle R. A review of 50 children with obstructive sleep apnea syndrome. *Lung* 1981; 159:275–287.

9. Wilkinson AR, McCormick MS, Freeland AP, Pickering D. Electrocardiographic signs of pulmonary hypertension in children who snore. *British Medical Jounal* 1981; 282:1579–1582.

10. Guilleminault C, ed. Obstructive sleep apnea syndrome in children. In *Sleep and Its Disorders in Children.* New York: Raven, 1987.

11. Guilleminault C, Ariagno R. Apnea during sleep in infants and children. In *Principles and Practice of Sleep Medicine.* Kryger MH, Roth T, Dement WC. Philadelphia: Saunders, 1989.

12. Lipton AJ, Gozal D. Treatment of obstructive sleep apnea in children: do we really know how? *Sleep Medicine Review* 7(1):61–80, 2003.

Chapter 14

1. Ball N. Personal communication, 2006.

2. Landis CA, Moe KE. Sleep and menopause. *Nursing Clinics of North America* 2004; 39:97–115.

3. Bixler EO, Vgontzas AN, Lin HM, et al. Prevalence of sleep-disordered breathing in women: effects of gender. *American Journal of Respiratory and Critical Care Medicine* 2001; 163:608–13.

4. Franklin KA, Holmgren PA, et al. Snoring, pregnancy-induced hypertension, and growth retardation of the fetus. *Chest* 2000; 117(1):137–141.

5. Santiago JR, Nolledo MS, Kinzler W, Santiago TV.. Sleep and sleep disorders in pregnancy. *Annals of Internal Medicine* 2001; 134:396–408.

6. Women and Sleep Poll, National *Sleep* Foundation, 1998.

7. Young T, Rabago D, Zigierska A, et al. Objective and subjective sleep quality in premenopausal, perimenopausal, and postmenopausal women in the Wisconsin sleep cohort study. Sleep 2003; 26(6):667–672.

Chapter 15

1. Prinz PN, Raskind M. Aging and sleep disorders. In *Sleep Disorders: Diagnosis and Treatment.* Williams RL, Karacan I. New York: Wiley, 1978.

2. Ancoli-Israel S, Kripke DF, Mason W, Kaplan OJ. Sleep apnea and periodic movements in an aging sample. *Journal of Gerontology* 1985; 40(4):419–425.

3. Carskadon M A, Dement WC. Respiration during sleep in the aged human. *Journal of Gerontology* 1981; 36(4):420–423.

4. Bliwise DL, Pascualy RA. Sleep-related respiratory disturbance in elderly persons. *Comprehensive Therapy* 1984; 10(7):8–14.

Chapter 18

1. Edinger JD, Radtke RA. Use of In vivo desensitization to treat a patient's claustrophobic response to nasal CPAP. *Sleep* 1993; 16(7):678–680.

Chapter 19

1. Dexter, D. Jr. Magnetic therapy is ineffective for the treatment of snoring and obstructive sleep apnea syndrome. *Wisconsin Medical Journal* 1997 Mar; 96(3):35–37.

Appendix

Addresses, Products, and Services for People with Sleep Apnea

The AWAKE Network: Sleep Apnea Support Groups

AWAKE is the national sleep apnea patient support network. There are AWAKE groups in every state and Canadian province. Your sleep center's CPAP coordinator should know about the nearest AWAKE group. If not, you can locate nearby AWAKE groups, or obtain guidelines on starting an AWAKE group, by contacting the American Sleep Apnea Association at sleepapnea.org.

American Sleep Apnea Association

The American Sleep Apnea Association (ASAA) is a national nonprofit organization dedicated to public and patient education and support for medical advances in sleep apnea. At the web site you can find a wealth of information on sleep apnea, AWAKE support groups in your area, CPAP equipment and support, and information on legal, workplace, and other issues affecting people with sleep apnea. They also have forums and live chats where you can interact with other sleep apnea folks.

American Sleep Apnea Association
Washington, DC 20005
Phone: 202-293-3650
FAX: 202-293-3656
sleepapnea.org

American Academy of Sleep Medicine

The American Academy of Sleep Medicine (AASM) (formerly the American Sleep Disorders Association, ASDA) is the professional sleep medicine organization that comprises individual members and accredited sleep centers and sleep laboratories.

You can find a list of all the accredited sleep centers in the United States and Canada on their web site at www.aasmnet.org by clicking on *Patients and Public* and then on *Find a sleep center* . Click on your state. When you have selected a sleep center from the list for your state, you can also find out whether that sleep center has board certified sleep medicine specialists on their staff. Look in the lower left corner of that sleep center page for the words: "Diplomats of the American Board of Sleep Medicine" which will be followed by a list of certified sleep medicine specialists at that sleep center (see below).

American Academy of Sleep Medicine
One Westbrook Corporate Center, Ste. 920,
Westchester, IL 60154
Phone (708) 492-0930
Fax: (708) 492-09431610

American Board of Sleep Medicine

The American Board of Sleep Medicine (ABSM), associated with the AASM, is the organization that establishes the standards of practice for sleep medicine, and issue accreditation in sleep medicine to physicians and PhDs who have earned this certificate through specialized study in this field. You can find a list of board certified sleep specialists at www.absm.org.

American Board of Sleep Medicine
One Westbrook Corporate Center, Ste 920
Westchester, Il 60154
Phone 708-492-1290
FAX 708-492-0943

National Sleep Foundation

The National Sleep Foundation (NSF) is a nonprofit organization whose mission is to improve the quality of life of people with sleep disorders, to increase public awareness of sleep issues, and to prevent catastrophic accidents related to sleep deprivation and disorders.

The NSF web site, www.sleepfoundation.org, has tons of excellent information about normal sleep and all of the sleep disorders, an "ask the expert" column, an opportunity to test your own sleep quality, and many other resources. The NSF publishes excellent brochures on each of the sleep disorders and other aspects of sleep.

Read their publication on sleep apnea on their web site. For a copy of their sleep apnea brochure, send your request and a self-addressed, stamped, business envelope to:

National Sleep Foundation
1522 K Street NW, Suite 500
Washington, D.C. 20005

American Academy of Dental Sleep Medicine

The American Academy of Dental Sleep Medicine (AADSM) is a professional membership organization promoting the use and research of oral appliances and oral surgery for the treatment of sleep apnea.

Their standards and certification arm, the American Board of Dental Sleep Medicine (ABDSM), tests and certifies dentists who have undertaken advanced study of sleep apnea and pass a qualifying exam.

For a list of dentists in your region who are familiar with the use of oral appliances for treating sleep apnea, go to their web site, www.dentalsleepmed.org, and click on *Patients*.

American Academy of Dental Sleep Medicine
One Westbrook Corporate Center, Suite 920
Westchester, IL 60154
Phone 708-273-9366
FAX 708-492-0943

Sleep Apnea on the Internet

Each of the above professional sleep medicine Internet sites has links to other sleep-related pages. In addition, below are two other reliable sites that are operated by bona fide medical organizations.

Sleepnet

Information, many links to other sleep sites, list of accredited sleep centers, forums, other resources, from Stanford School of Sleep Medicine.

www.sleepnet.com

The Sleep Home Pages

Great resource on current sleep medicine research.

www.sleephomepages.org/

Contacts for Other Sleep Disorders

Restless Legs/Periodic Limb Movement In Sleep (RLS/PLMS)

The RLS Foundation, www.rls.org, is a wonderful collaboration between patients, physicians, and researchers. Their newsletter, *Nightwalkers*, is first rate.

Narcolepsy

www.narcolepsynetwork.org
www.stanford.edu/~dement/narco.html

CPAP Manufacturers

Below are the major manufacturers of CPAP equipment and accessories as of 2007.

- ResMed Corp.
  14040 Danielson Street
  Poway CA 92064-6857
  San Diego, CA 92131
  800-424-0737
  www.resmed.com
- Respironics, Inc.
  1501 Ardmore Blvd.
  Pittsburgh, PA 15221-4401
  800-345-6643
  www.respironics.com

CPAP Equipment and Parts by Mail

You should not get your first CPAP by mail. It is best to begin your CPAP experience with a local durable medical equipment (DME) provider, where you should have an opportunity to try a variety of CPAP equipment, and should expect help, information, and support in getting started on CPAP.

However, in the future, depending on your satisfaction with the prices and service for your first CPAP, you may wish to explore other sources, including other local homecare providers.

The Internet is opening up the market for CPAP supplies such as filters, masks, headgear, and even replacement CPAPs, and prices are becoming more competitive—a welcome development for CPAP users.

Admittedly, the reason for the lower mail-order prices is that you do not receive the personal mask-fitting and trouble-shooting service that you should (but sometimes do not) receive from a local DME provider. You will be "on your own" and must be prepared to sacrifice service for lower prices.

The Internet source listed below is a favorite among CPAP users. You may find others. Compare prices and consider asking for references from other customers before buying.

The CPAP Store (Internet)

Started in 1997 by a CPAP user in his bedroom, this little Internet company sells equipment and supplies at 20 percent to 60 percent below retail. It has CPAP equipment and parts, tips, custom headgear, and fast service. Call or visit the web site for a price list.

7513 W. Kennewick Avenue, Suite D
Kennewick, WA 99336
Phone 509-735-1842
FAX (509) 735-1884
www.thecpapstore.com/

CPAP Supply USA (Internet)

Another internet CPAP store with a wide selection of items.

www.cpapsupplyusa.com/

Battery to Operate a CPAP Unit

A small, rechargeable, lithium ion battery came on the market in 2007. It is the size of a paperback book and weighs about 14 pounds. It comes with an assortment of adaptors and a plug for recharging from a car cigarette lighter. The number of hours it will run your CPAP unit depends on your pressure setting and other power demands of your machine. Some people will get more than one night's power from a single recharge. Great for travel "off the grid" if you have a vehicle for recharging, and as a backup power source in case of power failures.

However, before purchasing one of these batteries, you should check with your CPAP supplier or the manufacturer to make sure your CPAP unit will operate properly with this particular type of battery.

www.batterygeek.net

Some Common Drugs That Can Make Sleep Apnea Worse

Many medications can make sleep apnea worse by making you drowsy or by disturbing your sleep or breathing. Be sure to tell your sleep specialist about all of the medications you take, both over-the-counter and prescription drugs. The sleep specialist may want to adjust dosages or suggest alternatives.

Some common over-the-counter (nonprescription) drugs, such as antihistamines, can make sleep apnea worse. Ask your pharmacist about all nonprescription medications that you take frequently. Can they cause drowsiness, breathing problems, or insomnia? Can he suggest alternative medications with fewer side effects?

The following prescription drugs can cause problems for people with sleep apnea (Table A.1). (This is not a complete list.) If you are taking any of these drugs (or their generic form), or if you suspect that a medication may be affecting your sleep, be sure to discuss these matters with your sleep physician.

Drugs that Can Cause Drowsiness or Apnea or Insomnia			
	Drowsiness	Apnea	Insomnia
Actifed with Codeine Cough Syrup	xxx		
Alfenta		x	
Alferon N			xx
Ambien	xx		
Anafranil	xxx		
Anaprox, Anaprox DS	x		
Anestacon	xxx		
Asendin	xx		
Atgam		xx	
Atrofen	xxx		x
Benadryl	xxx		xxx
Bentyl	x		
Buspar	xx		x
Cardura	x		
Catapres, Catapres TTS	xxx		
Centrax	x		
CHEMET	xx		
Clozaril	xxx		
Combipres	xxx		
Cylert		xxx	

Continued

	Drowsiness	Apnea	Insomnia
Cytadren	xxx		
Dantrium	xxx		
Depo-Provera			x
Desyrel	xxx		x
DHC Plus	xxx		
Dilantin with Phenobarbital	xxx		
Doral	xx		
Duragesic	xx	xx	
Emcyt			x
Emete-con	xxx		
Empirin with Codeine	xxx		
Ergamisol	x		
Esgic-Plus	xxx		
Exosurf			xxx
Fioricet	xxx		
Fiorinal	xxx		
Flexeril	xxx		
Floxin			x
Habitrol	x		x
Halcion	xx		
Hismanal	x		
Hylorel	xx		
Hytrin	x		
IFEX	xxx		
Innovar		xxx	
Intron A	x	x	
Kerlone			x
Klonopin	xxx		
Limbitrol, Limbitrol DS	xxx		
Lioresal	xxx		x

Continued

	Drowsiness	Apnea	Insomnia
Lopressor HCT	xx		
Ludiomil	xx		
Lupron			x
Lysodren	xxx		
Marinol (Dronabinol)	xx		
Marplan	xxx		
Mazicon	x		
Mepron	xx		
Minipress	x		
Minizide	x		
Moban	xxx		
Nalfon 200	x		
Naprosyn	x		
Nicoderm			xx
Orudis			x
Parlodel	x		
Paxil	xx		xx
PedvaxHIB	xxx		
Permax	xx		x
Phenurone	x		
Phrenilin	xxx		
ProSom	xxx		
Prostep	x		x
Prostin VR		xx	
Prozac	xx		xx
Pyridium Plus	xxx		
Reglan	xx		
Restoril	xx		
Retrovir	x		x
Ritalin			xxx
Rynatan, Rynatan-S	xxx		
Rynatuss	xxx		

Continued

	Drowsiness	Apnea	Insomnia
Sanorex			xxx
Seconal	xxx		
Sectral			x
Sedapap	xxx		
Seldane, Seldane-D	x		xxx
Sinequan	xxx		
Soma, Soma with Codeine	xxx		
Stadol	xxx		xx
Suprane		xx	
Survanta		xxx	
Symmetrel	xx		
Synarel			x
Tavist, Tavist-1, Tavist-D	xxx		
Tegretol	xxx		
Temaril	xxx		x
Tenex	xxx		
Theo-X	xxx		
Toradol	x		xx
Trandate	x		
Transderm Scop	x		
Tranxene, Tranxene-SD	xxx		
Trinalin	xxx		
Tripedia	xx		
Valrelease	xxx		
Ventolin			x
Versed	xx		
Videx			xxx
Visken			xx
Wellbutrin			xx
Wytensin	xx		

Continued

	Drowsiness	Apnea	Insomnia
Xanax	xxx		xxx
Xylocaine	xxx		
Zoladex			x
Zoloft	xx		xx

The x's indicate the chances that a person taking the drug will experience the problem listed. (Based on data from *Physicians Desk Referencex*, 1993.)
x = small chance (problem affects fewer than 10% of people taking the drug)
xx = moderate chance (problem affects 10% to 25% of people taking the drug)
xxx = common problem (affects more than 25% of people taking the drug)

Glossary

Adenoids: Lymphoid tissue, similar to tonsils, but located behind and above the tonsils.

Airway: The passage through which air travels as it moves to and from your lungs; your airway includes nose and mouth, throat, and the bronchial tubes that lead to your lungs.

Angina pectoris: Chest pain that occurs when the heart muscle does not get enough oxygen.

Apnea: Failure to move air in and out of your airway.

Apnea event: Failure to breathe that lasts for more than 10 seconds.

Apnea index: The number of apnea events per hour; a measure of the severity of sleep apnea.

Apnea-plus-hypopnea index: The total number of apnea and hypopnea events per hour; a measure of the severity of sleep apnea.

Arrhythmia: Variation from the normal rhythm of the heartbeat.

Breathing center: The center in your brain that controls the speed and forcefulness of your breathing.

Carbon dioxide: The waste gas produced by your body; it is removed from your blood stream in the lungs and leaves the body when you exhale.

Cardiovascular: Pertaining to the heart or circulatory system.

Carotid body: A sensory structure in the carotid artery in the neck that measures the amount of oxygen in your blood and sends signals to the breathing center in your brain.

Central sleep apnea: Sleep apnea that is caused by some irregularity in the brain's control of breathing.

Cephalometry: Measurement of the size and location of the structures in the head using x-rays or other imaging systems.

Continuous positive airway pressure (CPAP): A breathing system used to treat obstructive sleep apnea and other respiratory disorders.

Cuirass: A breathing device that fits over a patient's chest and helps him or her breathe; sometimes used to treat central sleep apnea.

Deviated septum: An irregularly shaped nasal septum; may partly block the passage of air and interfere with breathing; see *nasal septum*.

Diaphragm: The muscular wall that separates the chest cavity from the abdominal cavity; your diaphragm is part of your breathing system; the downward contraction of the diaphragm muscles allows your lungs to expand and fill with air.

EDS: Excessive daytime sleepiness.

ENT specialist: Ear, nose, and throat specialist; also called an otolaryngologist.

Gastric bypass: A surgical procedure in which the stomach is stapled to make it smaller; used to promote weight loss in morbidly obese patients.

Hypertension: High blood pressure.

Hypopnea: Shallow breathing in which the airflow in and out of the airway is less than half of normal.

Larynx: The "voice box"; the structure in the lower throat that contains the vocal cords; the Adam's apple is the front of your larynx.

Laser-assisted uvulopalatoplasty (LAUP): laser surgery performed on the soft palate to reduce snoring; not recommended for sleep apnea.

Mandible: Lower jawbone.

Mandibular reconstruction: Surgery to reshape the lower jaw.

Maxilla: Upper jawbone.

Maxillofacial surgery: Surgery on the upper jaw and face.

Medulla oblongata: A deep, primitive part of the brain; sensors that detect carbon dioxide are located here; these sensors are involved in the breathing reflex.

Mixed sleep apnea: Sleep apnea that is a combination of obstructive and central apnea.

NREM sleep: Non-REM sleep; see *REM sleep*.

Nasal septum: The divider between the right and the left nose cavities; it is made up of bone, cartilage, and soft tissue.

Neurologic: Pertaining to the nervous system.

Nocturnal: Occurring at night.

Obese: Having a weight of more than 20% above the ideal body weight.

Obstructive sleep apnea: Sleep apnea caused by a blockage of the airway.

Oral pressure appliance (OPAP): A small mouthpiece that can be worn either by itself or connected to CPAP tubing and a CPAP machine.

Otolaryngologist: An ear, nose, and throat specialist; also called an ENT specialist.

Oxygen: A gas that makes up 20% of the air your breathe; it is picked up in your lungs by red blood cells and carried throughout your body; all your body's cells need oxygen in order to live.

Oxygen saturation: The amount of oxygen being carried in your blood; often used as a measure of the severity of sleep apnea; normal oxygen saturation is about 95%, with some decrease with age.

Pharynx: The part of the throat just behind the mouth.

Polycythemia: An abnormal excess of red blood cells.

Polysomnography: The recording of a person's breathing, heartbeat, brain activity, body movements, and other physiological signs during sleep.

Pulmonary: Pertaining to the lungs.

Red blood cells: The cells that carry oxygen through the bloodstream.

REM sleep: The "rapid eye movement" stage of sleep; the "active" stage of sleep during which the most vivid dreams occur.

Respiratory disturbance index (RDI): A measure of the severity of sleep apnea; equal to the number of apneas plus hypopneas, divided by total sleep time, and multiplied by 60.

Set point: The amount of carbon dioxide or oxygen in your blood that triggers the breathing center to make you inhale.

Sleep apnea: A condition in which a person stops breathing while asleep.

Sleep latency: The amount of time it takes for you to fall asleep; indicates the degree of excessive daytime sleepiness.

Soft palate: The flexible back part of the roof of your mouth.

Somnoplasty: A surgical technique for reducing snoring by using radio frequency energy.

Tonsils: A pair of small glands located at the back of the mouth, on either side of the opening into the throat.

Upper airway resistance syndrome (UARS): A type of sleep-disordered breathing associated with arousals from sleep; sometimes called respiratory effort–related arousals (RERAs)

Uvula: The dangling, tongue-shaped fleshy mass that hangs down from the soft palate at the back of your mouth.

Uvulopalatopharyngoplasty (UPPP): A type of surgery sometimes used to treat snoring and obstructive sleep apnea.

Index

CPSIA information can be obtained at www.ICGtesting.com
Printed in the USA
LVOW060743230613

339671LV00002B/94/P

9 781932 603262